David S. Bell
Mary Z. Robinson
Jean Pollard
Tom Robinson
Bonnie Floyd

A Parents' Guide to CFIDS
How to Be an Advocate for Your Child with Chronic Fatigue Immune Dysfunction

Pre-publication
REVIEWS,
COMMENTARIES,
EVALUATIONS . . .

"**D**r. Bell and colleagues offer insight and practical advice for parents of youngsters suffering from this poorly understood disease. It is clear from their writing that the authors have been in the trenches with this disorder and know its impacts firsthand. A nice balance is struck between offering advice on coping with the school system and the health care system on one hand and, on the other hand, suggestions for maintaining the spousal relationship and dealing with the impact of the disorder on the family.

The authors' caring, understanding, and commitment to children and adolescents with CFIDS clearly resound throughout the book.

This book is useful for parents of youngsters who have been recently diagnosed, as well as for those who have been plagued with the illness for years. Professionals working with YPWCs will also gain insight into the social and educational effects of CFIDS."

Karen M. Jordan, PhD
Adjunct Clinical Assistant Professor,
University of Illinois
at Chicago

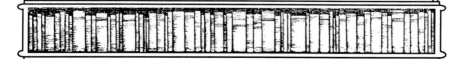

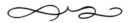
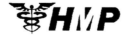

The Haworth Medical Press
An Imprint of The Haworth Press, Inc.

A Parents' Guide to CFIDS

How to Be an Advocate for Your Child with Chronic Fatigue Immune Dysfunction

A Parents' Guide to CFIDS
How to Be an Advocate for Your Child with Chronic Fatigue Immune Dysfunction

David S. Bell, MD, FAAP
Mary Z. Robinson, MSEd
Jean Pollard, AS
Tom Robinson, MS, CAS
Bonnie Floyd, MA

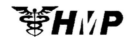

The Haworth Medical Press
An Imprint of The Haworth Press, Inc.
New York • London

Published by

The Haworth Medical Press®, an imprint of The Haworth Press, Inc., 10 Alice Street, Binghamton, NY 13904-1580

Cover design by Monica L. Seifert.

Illustration on p. vi by Libby Pollard.

Library of Congress Cataloging-in-Publication Data

A parents' guide to CFIDS : how to be an advocate for your child with chronic fatigue immune dysfunction syndrome / David S. Bell . . . [et al.].
    p.   cm.
Includes bibliographical references and index.
ISBN 0-7890-0711-8 (alk. paper)
    1. Chronic fatigue syndrome in children—Popular works. I. Bell, David S.
RJ381.P37 1999
616'.0478'083—dc21
                                           98-21756
                                             CIP

To all the YPWCs who struggle every day
with this illness.

My Life Is Drifting Away

by Megan, a seven-year-old YPWC

My life is drifting away.
It's all going to waste.
I do not show it, and I do not know it,
But all I can ask is when I'll be back home.
My family is looking and I took away the love,
Away from my family, away from me,
And away from our hearts.
My life is drifting away.

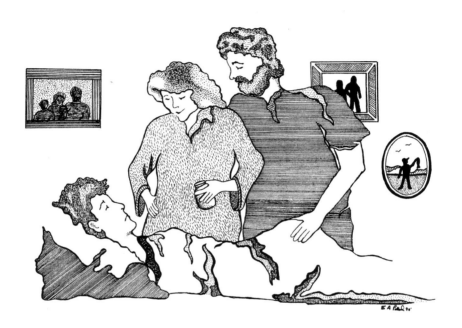

CONTENTS

ABOUT THE AUTHORS

David S. Bell, MD, a primary care physician in pediatrics and family practice, has been researching CFIDS since the outbreak in Lyndonville, New York, in 1985. He is a graduate of Harvard University and the Boston University School of Medicine. In addition to his private practice, he has also served as an instructor in pediatrics at both Harvard Medical School and the University of Rochester and as a consultant in clinical immunology at the State University of New York at Buffalo. Dr. Bell has been involved in the clinical research of Chronic Fatigue Immune Dysfunction Syndrome, with a special interest in children afflicted with this illness. He has a number of credits to his name, including advisory appointments to a variety of CFIDS journals and organizations. He has spoken at dozens of conferences and lectures around the world on CFIDS research and has an extensive amount of journal and medical publications to his name. He is the author of two books on CFIDS, *The Disease of a Thousand Names,* published in 1991; and *The Doctor's Guide to Chronic Fatigue Syndrome,* published in 1994.

Jean Pollard, AS, lives in Lyndonville, New York, with her husband, Paul. She is a graduate of the Rochester Institute of Technology and has worked for Dr. David S. Bell as his personal secretary and office manager for the past seventeen years. In 1990, she published Dr. Bell's first book titled *The Disease of a Thousand Names.* She became involved in CFIDS when all four of her children developed this illness in November 1985. These were Dr. Bell's first CFIDS patients. Jean has spent the last twelve years dedicating herself to the tasks of researching this illness, as Dr. Bell's research assistant, helping patients to live and cope with this illness, and educating the public through magazine and television interviews on both local and national TV.

Tom and Mary Robinson have been married for sixteen years and reside in Medina, New York, with their three children. Their oldest child, a fourteen-year-old boy, has had CFIDS for four years, and their seven-year-old daughter was stricken at age five. Their middle daughter shows no signs of the illness. Struggling to face the obstacles of parenting two YPWCs, Tom and Mary started the Medina Area CFIDS Youth Support Group for Children with CFIDS and Their Families.

Mary earned her BS and MS degrees in education from SUNY College at Oswego. Although an elementary teacher by training, she is a stay-at-home mother by choice. She is a research assistant for Dr. Bell. In addition to contributing to many of the chapters, Mary also had the tedious task of editing and compiling all the chapters into book form.

Tom earned his BA degree in psychology at LeMoyne College in Syracuse and his MS degree and CAS in the School of Counseling at SUNY College at Oswego. He has been a School Counselor for eighteen years and has served on the Committee on Special Education (CSE) for most of that time.

Bonnie Floyd earned a BS degree in psychology at SUNY at Brockport and a MA degree in psychology, with a behavioral medicine concentration, at Connecticut College. Her MA thesis was "Psychosocial Adaptation to Chronic Fatigue Syndrome." She is currently a doctoral student in the Clinical Health Psychology program at Yeshiva University, Ferkauf Graduate School of Psychology, and the Albert Einstein College of Medicine.

Acknowledgments

Our deepest gratitude goes to Cynthia Holzafhel of The Book Publishing Company for reviewing our manuscript and offering ideas on how to proceed with the task of producing a book. Cynthia was always there to offer ideas, perspectives, and a fresh approach to the task of editing.

Our sincere appreciation goes to Kate Anderson, MEd, from British Columbia, Canada, for helping us with the final edit of the book. Kate's main contribution was to Chapter 6, which she helped us to rewrite. Kate has suffered from CFIDS for over ten years and has recently become more aware of the special challenges facing children and adolescents with CFIDS. In addition to working on her doctorate, Kate also works out of her home as a distance education instructor in Child and Youth Care and as a parent educator, specializing in helping parents deal with temperament differences in their children.

We offer thanks to Bruce Goldstein, who is an attorney in Buffalo, New York, specializing in disability law, for assisting us in citations of the law and for clarifying some questions on these laws. He is the co-author of a book titled *Legal Rights of Persons with Disabilities: An Analysis of Federal Law* (1991).

Finally, thanks go to our friends and families, who offered unwavering support, encouragement, and feedback on the manuscript in terms of content and editing. We never would have completed this book without each one of you. Our thanks to you all!

Introduction

When chronic fatigue immune dysfunction syndrome (CFIDS) appears in childhood, it presents many physical, social, emotional, and academic challenges. CFIDS, which is also known as chronic fatigue syndrome (CFS), fibromyalgia (FM), or myalgic encephalomyelitis (ME), is one of the most complicated illnesses in the history of medicine. It is easy to see why parents may have difficulty understanding this disease and become discouraged, believing that they do not know enough about their child's medical problems. Most doctors do not even understand the illness. Becoming informed about CFIDS can make the road to understanding and helping your child much easier to travel. Some parents may feel guilty about their child becoming ill, especially if they themselves have CFIDS. There is nothing any parent can do to prevent it. Parents who cope with these troubling feelings are taking the first step toward acceptance and being able to support their child.

This book was designed with several goals in mind. It is meant as a guide for parents and educators involved in developing the best academic program for the Young Person with CFIDS (YPWC). The consensus of the authors is that developing a positive working relationship with school personnel is critical to the success of any accommodations made for the student's education. The beginning work on this book revealed that the parents' role in dealing with a sick child must also be addressed. Learning how to communicate and function, not only with the outside world, but also within your family, is of key importance in getting your child the help he or she needs. This, at times, can be a more difficult job than working with the school.

Within the school, ongoing communication throughout the year is important both for the parent and for the teachers or other school liaisons. The best situation is one in which the parents and the school personnel form a partnership. They must work together to develop and implement the best educational plan possible, keeping in mind that flexibility is the key to success.

The academic challenges of CFIDS are major hurdles to overcome. Even more difficult, though, are the social challenges CFIDS inflicts on these individuals. YPWCs are cut off from their friends and peers at a critical stage of self-development. Socialization for the normal child and the YPWC is discussed throughout the book from the perspectives of adults and parents, as well as from those of teenagers suffering from CFIDS.

It is our hope that this book will provide you with the tools needed to build positive relationships with your family, physicians, and the educators at your child's school. Better understanding of the challenges that your child faces and the educational modifications available will prepare you to assist your youngster in obtaining the best education possible. As a parent, you must love your child, first and foremost. You must trust and believe in your child. *You* are your child's number one advocate to everyone, from the medical community to the school, from family to friends. You are this child's advocate in life.

In June 1996, we met for the first time to discuss educational planning for the YPWC. At this meeting, the educators shared with Dr. Bell and his office manager, Jean Pollard, the issues the school encounters when faced with a child with CFIDS. We attempted to at least open some doors and begin to foster an understanding of how doctors can assist in the educational planning for these children. Dr. Bell suggested that with the wealth of information being shared, we could present it in a usable form for parents who were desperate for information on educating their children. On that night, this book was born.

PERSONAL ISSUES
SURROUNDING CFIDS

Chapter 1

How Do You Know If Your Child Has CFIDS?

THE SYMPTOMS

If you have picked up a copy of this book, your child has probably been diagnosed by a health professional as having chronic fatigue immune dysfunction syndrome (CFIDS.) Although you may have spent some time learning about the symptoms and effects of this illness, it will help both you and your child to understand how varied these symptoms can be. What your child may be currently feeling can change over time. It may also be comforting to know that what your child is experiencing is not unique: this puzzling combination of discomforts and complaints is common to both adults and children who are struggling with this illness.

For young persons with CFIDS (YPWCs), exhaustion is the most common complaint, just as it is for adults with CFIDS. They may not look as sick as they say they are; although at times they may look pale, or at other times flushed. For the most part, they will look like normal, healthy children. However, as time goes on, you and other adults with whom your child has regular contact (teachers, the school nurse, or home tutor) will begin to see a relationship between how your child feels and how he or she appears.

For example, when the illness becomes more severe, your child will become increasingly tired. Along with this exhaustion, your child can experience, or exhibit, many other symptoms:

- Dizziness
- Light-headedness
- Fainting spells
- Headache
- Abdominal pain

- Lack of restful sleep and insomnia
- Night sweats
- Sore throat
- Lymph node pain
- Short-term memory loss
- Inability to concentrate
- Muscle and joint pain
- Eye pain
- Light sensitivity
- Flushing and rashes on the face and neck
- Fever and chills
- Numbness and tingling in the fingers and toes
- Allergies and chemical sensitivities
- Diarrhea
- Constipation
- Weight gain
- Panic attacks
- Shortness of breath
- Palpitations

This list may seem daunting, but many of these symptoms are what you would experience with the onset of the flu. The fatigue is a completely overwhelming, aching discomfort that tends to occur along with other symptoms, such as sore throat or stomach pain. Diagnosing CFIDS is frustrating because nearly all of us have had these symptoms at one time or another. What makes CFIDS so unusual is that this pattern of symptoms can last for months, or even years.

It is also important to remember that although fatigue may be the most common symptom of CFIDS, it may not be the worst symptom your child experiences. In a group of 100 CFIDS patients, half reported that fatigue was their biggest problem; however, the other half felt that they suffered more from their inability to concentrate, headaches, muscle pain, sore throats, lymph node pain, abdominal pain, joint pains, and other discomforts. Doctors must remember the *pattern* of the symptoms when diagnosing CFIDS. If CFIDS were a patchwork quilt, each symptom would be a different color. In any person, one color may dominate, making that quilt look different from the others. One person might have a quilt that has more blue patches, another's quilt might have more red, but the overall pattern is the same. To diagnose CFIDS is to see the overall appearance of the quilt and not focus on any one color.

Another way of looking at CFIDS is to divide your child's symptoms into specific groups, putting more emphasis on the pattern of symptoms rather than labeling one specific symptom as more important than another. For example, abdominal pain may be a minor symptom for one child, but the most severe symptom for another. Your child may have more symptoms from one group than another, but he or she will have symptoms in each group, and that will be the most significant way to diagnose the illness. The symptoms fall into four basic categories: fatigue, pain, cognitive and neurological difficulties (how we learn, think, and remember, and how our senses operate), and sensitivities to various substances.

Fatigue

The word "fatigue" does not really describe the debilitating exhaustion that characterizes CFIDS. Instead, it implies a sensation with which we are all familiar—being tired after a long day. The fatigue of CFIDS, however, is an exhaustion that is combined with malaise or a flulike feeling, weakness, and a sensation of impending total collapse. With the fatigue of a hard day, it is possible to push through and keep on going—a sensation all parents feel after being up all night with a new baby or sick child. With CFIDS fatigue, it is impossible to stay awake and continue working; the only option is to lie down and rest. In fact, this weakness is nearly always more pronounced when the YPWC is standing or sitting up.

Fatigue is the most limiting symptom of CFIDS. At its most severe, it is characterized by a constant malaise or feeling of illness. In its milder form, the malaise weakens into tiredness. It is only during this milder phase that it is possible for an individual to "push through" the fatigue and keep on going, as is typical of the fatigue of everyday life.

The most distinctive aspect of CFIDS fatigue is that it worsens after exertion. In fact, this can be one way to determine whether your child has CFIDS. A child who feels good while spending a few hours in school or playing with a friend, but is exhausted for a whole day afterward is exhibiting typical CFIDS symptoms. With most other illnesses associated with fatigue, sufferers will tend to be exhausted while they try to do something, not afterward.

Pain

The second group of CFIDS symptoms is pain. CFIDS pain can be felt in most areas of the body: muscles, joints, throat, lymph nodes, stomach, and head. The muscle pain is a general aching in the large muscles in the legs, arms, back, and sometimes the chest. At times, the pain is sharp in these specific areas. To touch or put pressure on these points triggers a cry of pain from the sufferer and thus they have come to be known as "trigger points." The joint pain appears in both the large and small joints, may move around—one minute the fingers, then the ankle, and in an hour, the knee—and is often thought of as growing pains. The headaches may be of several types, but frequently are considered migraines. With CFIDS, a sore throat is usually scratchy, and lymph glands are often sore in the neck and armpits. Your child can be experiencing pain in many places at the same time, yet because every test performed on these areas comes up negative, it can be very frustrating for the doctor, you, and your child. Teachers at school will find it difficult to believe that your child suffers so severely while looking so healthy. However, if you have ever been around someone with a migraine, you know what it is like to see someone suffering intense pain without being able to sense the severity of that pain.

Cognitive and Neurological Difficulties

The most dominant neurological problems that YPWCs experience, which affect them the most in school, are the cognitive problems associated with CFIDS, including short-term memory loss, forgetfulness, and a short attention span. (Teenagers, with their characteristic flair for description, call these symptoms "brain fog" or "brain sludge," because of how difficult it is for them to process information and pay attention to what they are doing.) Neurological problems your child might experience include numbness and tingling, clumsiness, dizziness, light-headedness, and loss of balance. These problems are usually either fleeting or not severe enough to limit your child's daily routine.

To give you a clearer idea of how CFIDS affects the functioning of a young person's brain, imagine two healthy young people who have been out all night dancing. In the morning, their fatigue will make it more difficult for them to focus their attention and process information. Given a good rest, however, they will be able to concentrate and learn at their usual level. For YPWCs, no amount of rest seems to correct this problem.

Children may complain that they do not remember what they read as well as they did before they were sick. Again, this is a frustrating aspect of the disease because you do not always have a good measure of how well these children retained information before developing CFIDS. They also will find it more difficult to "do two things at once," which is known in education as "multitasking." One of the hallmarks of a healthy teenager is the ability to listen to the radio, talk on the telephone, and do homework, all at the same time. With CFIDS, YPWCs could be driving home and get lost near their own driveway. Since much of the information we use to orient ourselves in our daily tasks is subtle and subconscious, we are often unaware of storing it. A CFIDS sufferer seems to have more problems than most people do in summoning up these subconscious cues.

Sensitivities

The fourth group of symptoms is sensitivities, which, although helpful in identifying CFIDS, usually are not severe. Your child may have unusual sensitivities to many things, such as light, odors, and noise. For instance, being in a large school lunchroom with fluorescent lights and a lot of noise may be very difficult for your YPWC. Some YPWCs experience eye discomfort and light sensitivity, and it is not uncommon to see them wearing sunglasses indoors. In addition, these sensitivities are likely to make your child's fatigue and other symptoms worse. In general, YPWCs are able to accurately describe the degrees of sensitivity they have. They may find that taking tests in classrooms with fluorescent lighting and/or echoing noises may be very difficult. If so, you can request educational accommodations, such as testing modifications and taking tests in alternate locations with natural lighting.

Patients with CFIDS are also unusually sensitive to drugs, and many will have multiple allergies. Alcohol sensitivity is very frequent, and any adolescent who regularly drinks alcohol is unlikely to have CFIDS.

DIFFERENCES BETWEEN CHILDREN AND ADULTS WITH CFIDS

Much more attention has been given to adults with CFIDS than to the children who suffer. Although CFIDS can have the same effect on both adults and children, children often react to its symptoms differently. Regarding fatigue, adults have had many years of experience with their energy levels. When normal patterns are disrupted, they are aware of it immediately. Because children (especially young children) are growing so fast, they are not as good at recognizing a change in their endurance. The same thing is true of cognitive changes. Although adults are used to the way they think, remember, and solve problems, children are still developing these skills. They are not able to explain what they are going through. But as a parent, you may be aware that your child just is not the same. A minor, but interesting, difference between adults with CFIDS and YPWCs is the facial flushing that occurs with children. YPWCs will sometimes look pale, then become extremely flushed, as if embarrassed. (It is this prominent flush that sometimes causes observers to comment on how healthy your child appears.)

INACCURATE DIAGNOSES

One of the most frustrating aspects of CFIDS is how often it is confused with emotional illness. A child who is fatigued much of the time without an obvious physical reason is typically diagnosed as depressed. Childhood depression is very real, but it is accompanied by feelings of hopelessness, despair, or sadness. A child with CFIDS may be discouraged about being sick, but his or her outlook on life is usually not desperate. The fatigue of CFIDS is different from the fatigue of depression. Depression is associated with apathy, lack of motivation, and lethargy and is improved by exertion and exercise. YPWCs want to be active but feel worse after such exertion. Both children with CFIDS and those with depression suffer from sleep disturbances and cognitive problems, but the nature of these problems will not be the same in both instances. For example, sleep disturbance in depression involves early awakening, while in CFIDS, it is sleep phase reversal. In terms of cognitive problems in depression, they tend to be a general slowing of the cognitive process, while in CFIDS, they are manifested as difficulty maintaining focus and attention. Also, CFIDS includes other symptoms such as fever, joint and muscle pain, tender lymph nodes, sore throats, and sensitivities that are not found with depression. Because of their difficulties attending school, children with CFIDS are often misdiagnosed as being "school phobic." Children who are truly school phobic develop symptoms designed to avoid school, but usually feel better during afternoons and weekends when school is out. YPWCs want to go to school and often feel worse on the weekends because of the exertion from attending classes.

In rare cases, some doctors may believe that the parents themselves are causing their children's CFIDS symptoms. "Munchausen syndrome by proxy" is a term describing an illness created by a parent that involves an active deception or fabrication of symptoms. A parent gains some sort of emotional fulfillment when his or her child is ill, so the parent will cause the child's symptoms. Because the parent of a child with CFIDS is so often the child's advocate with doctors, and because the illness is difficult for some doctors to diagnose, the parent might be suspected of "creating" the symptoms. In any event, it is helpful for the doctor to hear about the symptoms directly from your child. Sometimes he or she will mention things in a doctor's office of which you were unaware.

Since YPWCs are often assumed to be suffering from an emotional illness, it is important to know the specific symptoms that make CFIDS unique. Until we have a conclusive test for CFIDS, and until more physicians understand CFIDS symptoms, parents of YPWCs must play a special role in supporting their youngsters and helping others understand their children's needs. A health questionnaire that has been developed and used by school personnel to document evidence of CFIDS is included in the appendixes of this book (see Appendix A).

Chapter 2

CFIDS:
The Misunderstood Illness

The problems involved with getting people to realize that your child has CFIDS are almost as difficult as coping with the illness itself. Perhaps more than with any other illness existing today, CFIDS is extremely difficult for the average family physician (and specialist) to diagnose. And certainly, it is unlike any illness most parents will ever come up against. The fact that your child feels so ill, yet no one can seem to find a reason why, intensifies the difficulties your child faces. The doubts created by the inability to diagnose the problem arises from the "CFIDS dilemma."

When your child first becomes ill, it is typical for you, as parents, to have reservations. Your child looks well, yet complains constantly. Your doctor will probably say there is nothing wrong. Sometimes you will notice that there is a day or two when your child seems fairly normal, such as a day roller skating with friends. With an injury or illness such as a broken bone or cancer, this occasional good day is not possible. Therefore, you develop your own doubts. How can your child's illness be physical with so many erratic symptoms and days?

Your child will immediately sense your doubt—"You don't believe me!"—which places you in a difficult position. Your doctor may insist that there is nothing wrong, that you should send your child back to school and discourage complaints about imaginary symptoms. Many fathers take the bold, strong stance: "There is nothing wrong with my child." Yet, even as they say this, they may feel instinctively that this still is not the answer—all the pieces do not quite fit. Mothers usually take a protective position: "My child is sick and just needs rest." The stage is now set for a family argument, and the dilemma expands. Not only does your child feel ill, but he or she is also the cause of family arguments; and since nothing can be done to resolve this conflict, the child feels extremely helpless.

Then there is the doctor who is treating your child. No matter how many symptoms your child complains about, your doctor will most likely be unable to give you any reason for them. Physical examinations and lab tests will show nothing. Faced with this situation, your doctor will probably conclude that nothing is wrong and that some unknown psychological problem is causing your child to fabricate his or her illness. To the doctor, this makes sense. Your child's activity is severely limited and his or her inability to do things is similar to the condition of someone in the terminal stages of illnesses such as cancer and AIDS. Consequently, your doctor is unwilling to believe that a physical cause exists, since he or she cannot detect one with either tests or examinations. Although not fully understood, CFIDS does cause an activity limitation that can be severe, and this limitation occurs despite your child's healthy appearance and normal results from routine blood tests.

Finally, both you and your child must face the dilemma of school. If your child suffers from so much pain and exhaustion that simply taking a shower and getting dressed is an ordeal, then regular school attendance is not possible. The school will notice these absences and insist on an explanation. Since your doctor will be unable to provide a satisfactory answer, the school will suspect truancy. Continual absence might lead them to contact social services. If social services agrees with the doctor that no compelling reason exists for your child to miss school, they may initiate legal action against you.

Another important matter to consider is your child's relationships with friends. As with many YPWCs, your child will probably try to hide the symptoms from friends for as long as possible, joining activities whenever he or she feels up to it. When YPWCs reach the point when they can no longer hide that they are too exhausted to keep up, they will tend to withdraw from their circle of friends. Children, especially teenagers, have such a great need to fit in, to be like everyone else, that the stigma of constantly being sick can embarrass them. The desire to keep their illness a secret brings about feelings of guilt and shame that only cause them to withdraw even more from their social lives.

The CFIDS dilemma can seem a hopeless cycle—because CFIDS is not understood, it must not exist. Children's illnesses should not be attributed to anything such as child abuse, emotional problems, or malingering merely because their symptoms cannot be explained. Actually, other ailments are also difficult to diagnose, such as polio, head injuries, and certain types of poisonings. A polio virus infection can cause severe fatigue and symptoms remarkably similar to CFIDS, yet a routine physical exam or lab testing will not reveal anything conclusive.

The basis of CFIDS is a real medical or organic insult or injury. Steady but slow progress is being made toward uncovering the cause. Until this becomes known, children with CFIDS will continue to face the medical, social, and educational dilemmas of this illness. Remarkably, they tend to do so with a courage unknown to the healthy adults who judge them.

Chapter 3

How to Balance Your Family Life When You Have a Child with CFIDS

Do you ever feel as if you are alone on a roller coaster? That is how many parents of YPWCs describe their lives. A normal day here, a bedridden one the next. It is enough to make any parent feel crazy and to leave any family feeling constantly disrupted. The act of having to continually *live for the moment* is very unsettling, but it can be done.

When facing the many issues surrounding CFIDS, you may find yourself becoming easily discouraged. However, although daily problems may challenge your family, small triumphs will also occur, and families must make enjoying these good times a priority. CFIDS is an illness with constant relapses and remissions, and it makes daily life a constant trial. It is not at all uncommon for your child to experience remission and feel great for days, weeks, or maybe even months, and it is difficult for everyone when and if the relapse occurs. How do we allow ourselves to enjoy the good days when we do not know how long they will last? Must we always be prepared for the relapses? Some say that this is equivalent to living life under a dark cloud. In our experience, to combat this feeling, you must remember not to become discouraged when your children suffer relapses, and also not to become overconfident when they are in remission. Developing a false sense of security is easy. Allow yourself time to catch your breath during these good times, but also be prepared for the fall if they do not last.

You may find yourself becoming despondent over these relapses. This is normal, and there may be no way to avoid it. We too have felt overwhelmed with it all, even those of us who have been coping with CFIDS for years. We have found support in others and in places where we can talk freely about our own issues, which is critical to our daily survival. As parents, we are expected to overcome many monumental problems during the course of this illness. Some will occur within the family, many are at the school level, and as our children grow, different social issues arise. As the mother of four children with CFIDS advises, "Take one day at a time. I know that this sounds cliché, but it's true. And above all else, keep your sense of humor."

We have found support groups to be an important means of dealing with all the issues that arise. These groups offer companionship, knowledge, and coping skills, and many people benefit from interacting with others who face similar situations. Both national and local support groups exist (see Appendix B), and these groups have many different focuses: groups for YPWCs, general CFIDS groups, caregivers, parents—the list goes on. It is important to find a group that addresses your needs. If no local group exists in your area, you might consider forming one with other families suffering the same frustrations.

Another avenue for support is pen pals (see Appendix B— National Organizations). These programs match YPWCs to each other, healthy siblings to healthy siblings, and parents to parents. As one mother stated, "It's like a support group through the mail. When I get letters from my pen pals, I know exactly what they're feeling and going through. And when I'm feeling all alone and overwhelmed, I know I can write to them and they'll really understand."

Other YPWCs enjoy what they call "phone pals." These may be other YPWCs or any friends with whom they can stay in touch via the telephone. Even parents can get the support they need by picking up the phone and talking to someone who understands, helping them to feel less isolated and more in touch with the outside world.

Another type of support is available for those families owning home computers and having access to on-line services. A tremendous network is out there for children and adults alike. Children can go on-line and talk to others in the same situation. Parents can attend support groups for caregivers of PWCs, and they can join e-mail support groups or CFIDS newsgroups, without going farther than their computer. There are also dozens of informational sites on the World Wide Web with a wealth of information on CFIDS and related disorders. A new frontier is opening up and expanding quickly, and many are happy they investigated it. (See Appendix C for on-line resources.)

THE YPWC

Parenting a child with CFIDS is a heart-wrenching situation for anyone. Watching your child suffer through the days and nights can become a physical and emotional strain on the entire family. You may find yourself compensating for your child's illness by over-dosing him or her with attention and extra privileges that would never be offered if he or she was healthy. Although there is nothing wrong with extra attention and affection at certain times, if given too frequently, it can also lead to fear and more problems. Your child may actually become more worried, questioning why Mom and/or Dad are being so nice. This may result in increased anxiety that is unrelated to the illness. The situation is even more difficult when your child does not understand or know how to cope with this added attention.

For this reason, YPWCs do better when treated as normally as possible. They need to be able to put their illness in perspective and not allow it to take over their lives. This is true even though they may be very ill, perhaps bedridden, or just having a difficult time with symptoms. YPWCs must have some stability in their environment. Having a routine to rely on, when possible, helps them to maintain some control in their lives. Simple activities such as keeping a clean room, making their bed, and brushing their teeth are all parts of basic personal hygiene for which they should be held responsible. YPWCs should have chores, just as other family members do, that are tailored to their ability to perform such tasks. For one child, it may be doing the dishes, for another, sorting and rolling the socks. Children are extremely adaptable and resilient when given the opportunity.

We encourage and expect each of our children to be as much a part of family activities such as outings and parties as he or she can. A drive on a pleasant autumn day to see the changing leaves can be a very rewarding and memorable experience for the entire family. Some YPWCs have felt safer avoiding all outside contact for fear of rejection or to escape facing others' disbelief regarding their illness. This is unfortunate because being a part of the family and feeling needed is very important to these children. In addition to family togetherness, YPWCs can also benefit from support networks, as mentioned in the parents' section later in this chapter. Support groups, pen pals, even individual visits with a counselor can help to sort out problems and issues with which your child may be struggling. We found that when our children really felt loved and accepted for who they were, it became far easier for them to cope with the many challenges they faced.

THE SPECIAL PROBLEMS OF BEING A BROTHER OR SISTER OF A YPWC

Even in an average home, the normal give-and-take between children can present challenges to parenting skills. When one, or more, of the children becomes ill with a chronic condition such as CFIDS, the challenges are intensified. Brothers or sisters may take out their own feelings of frustration and jealousy on their ill sibling. They may not understand why this child is getting all the attention. Even if they do understand, they still have many conflicting feelings and emotions that are a source of confusion to them. Although their needs must also be attended to, they should not be allowed to make light of their sibling's illness. At the same time, YPWCs should be expected to act appropriately. Just because they are ill does not give them the right to act out or be inconsiderate of others in the family. The difficult task parents face is to try to determine what is a normal interaction between siblings and what is inappropriate behavior. Siblings need to learn the normal give-and-take of living with others, and they should be allowed that interaction with the least interference possible from parents. Sometimes it just helps to remind each child of how others are feeling.

Family meetings can be a good way to discuss all that is happening in your family. To be most effective, everyone in your family should be included in these discussions. While addressing the issues of the YPWC, parents must also remember that healthy children have needs apart from those of their sick sibling(s). We have tried to maintain a healthy family life by spending time with each of our children individually, as well as together. One father goes to work a half hour later one day a week so that he can drive his daughter to school on that day. One mother rises a half hour earlier to spend time alone with her healthy child, talking, reading, or just being together.

If you have several children with CFIDS, it is not always easy to give each of the children the attention he or she craves. At times, meeting the needs of any healthy youngsters you might have is even more difficult.

"I always feel like there's someone who needs me, and I can't be there. They each need 100 percent of me, and no matter how hard I juggle, someone is always getting shortchanged," remarked one YPWC's mother.

Your healthy children may have psychological issues that need to be addressed. Maybe they do not want to burden you with problems they think are small in comparison to the problems of their sick sibling(s). Finding someone outside your family with whom your children can share concerns is often helpful. This may lead your children to be more open in sharing their feelings and frustrations. This person may be a favorite teacher, a school counselor, or a professional counselor/psychologist who understands your family's situation. Some issues that could possibly be addressed are the fear of getting sick, the guilt about being healthy, and the thought that they contributed in some way to their brother or sister becoming ill. They may also need to discuss the grief they feel over the loss of a playmate. Other difficulties faced by siblings of YPWCs include having to get up each morning for school while the YPWC is still asleep, being at school knowing their sibling is home, and feeling jealous because the YPWC gets more attention from you, their grandparents, and friends of the family. This jealousy, in turn, may produce more feelings of guilt.

In one family, the YPWC stated that her siblings thought she was faking it for the many years that she was ill. Being the youngest child, they believed she was spoiled and taking advantage of their parents' attention. Her parents stated:

> When we made it a priority to spend time alone with our healthy children, we found it made a big difference in their ability to cope with the family circumstances. Reading with them, talking over their day, or going out for breakfast or lunch are all things that didn't require a large time commitment. However, these activities can make a world of difference to a child of any age.

Your healthy child may need help developing interests outside of the home. Many activities are available for children these days, and finding one your children want to participate in should not be difficult. Life can even get a bit hectic running children to and from dance classes, piano lessons, baseball practices, and other activities. Carpooling can be arranged with others in the class/activity if driving is a problem, or you can hire young adults to do the driving. No matter what the activity, it is important for your healthy children to have normal, active lives.

Attending or helping out at school functions, such as open houses, school performances, or class parties, can also be rewarding experiences for all, even if we have had to arrange for child care for our ill children. Such personal attention to your healthy child helps maintain a sense of balance in the family. Parents who are ill themselves and housebound can have someone tape the events they cannot attend. They can then take time to watch the tape, possibly with the child. In this way, the parent can still partake in the event. Sharing the event with the child and showing an interest in his or her activities is extremely important.

YOUR CHANGING ROLE AS A PARENT OF A YPWC

This section is devoted to you, the parent. Although we will refer to "parents" in this section, this term could denote any caregiver—a mother or father and significant other, a stepparent, a single parent, or even a grandparent—anyone serving as your child's advocate.

People approach illness and crises differently. Some face difficulties head on, while others prefer to avoid thinking about the problems. In most relationships, the two parents play different roles, and these roles become more defined as children enter the family. Many families seem to share certain dynamics. Some believe a basic biological difference makes the relationship between a father and his child different from that of a mother and her child. Most of the time, a child feels more comfortable snuggling and cuddling with Mom, and tumbling and rumbling with Dad. Children grow up seeking comfort from Mother's arms and reassurance that the world is OK from Dad.

What happens to the family when Mom's arms can no longer heal all the ills of the world and Dad cannot reassure the child that indeed the world is safe? Herein lies another dilemma of the CFIDS story, one that cannot be easily resolved. When the stress of having a sick child invades your family, all the dynamics change. When one parent becomes the primary caregiver, the other may benefit by making a special effort to develop a stronger relationship with the child than he or she previously had. For YPWCs who cannot do the things they used to do, such as football, baseball, camping, dancing, or biking, finding new activities in which they can participate is essential. Some activities that we find enjoyable are watching movies, going shopping, reading together, playing simple games, going out for ice cream or cocoa, or just listening to music. Some YPWCs are able to tolerate certain normal activities with minor changes. Basketball, with frequent rest breaks, is an option for some; others can handle golf, if using a golf cart. Activities that can accommodate rest breaks and vary energy expenditure are best. No matter what the activity, being together is a tremendous benefit to both your YPWC and you.

A Father's Special Challenge

Many times the mother becomes the child's protector, trying to shelter her YPWC from the harsh realities of illness. She may pamper her child, or at least her actions are seen as pampering by some. In reality, she may be the only one who believes that her child is physically ill. The father may notice this pampering and fear that too much coddling will remove the child's incentive to get well. He may then decide it is time for his child to reenter the world and push the YPWC to return to normal activities—to attend school, social activities, sports, and so on. The mother does not understand why the father is insisting their child engage in activities that he or she is obviously too ill to do. The father believes that if someone does not take control of this situation, their child may never be able to return to normal.

Depending on the situation, a variety of things may happen. The mother may react harshly to the father for his apparent insensitivity, and he may retreat to work, outside activities, or anything that keeps him from having to deal with the problem at hand—his sick child. He may feel totally helpless, being unable to do what he has always done—make the world OK. In another case, the father may try to control the situation by calling all the shots. This usually results in disharmony among all involved, and ultimately, the child begins to think: "Dad doesn't believe me."

The fathers we discussed this with agreed:

> One male trait that is very common is the need for fathers to maintain control, to fix situations. If your child has a broken arm, you make sure that he or she gets the necessary medical care by getting to the emergency room, ensuring proper care, and seeing that the bills get paid. Such nurturing is quite different from that of your wife, whose role is to provide emotional support while the ordeal is going on. With CFIDS, it's difficult to play out your usual role as a father. Some physicians say there is nothing wrong; therefore, you cannot arrange medical care. There is no exercise or activity you can provide to cure this problem. Sometimes, in a state of helplessness, you may even become angry, sometimes even agreeing with the physician that there is nothing wrong. If fathers are not able to fix the situation, some may deny that the situation needs fixing.
>
> The solution is to step back and listen. Put aside the impulse to "do." You are not able to correct this illness any more than physicians are, but as a father, you should be able to listen to and understand the feelings of your child. Being emotionally supportive is not going to make the illness worse.

As a child/parents' support group leader stated, "Something I hear in practically every call from a mother is that *the father just can't accept this,* and she has no idea why he is refusing to try to understand."

One reason may be that many fathers tend to be the "strong, silent type," and they often have difficulty sharing their feelings of anguish over their children's illness. Although this is normal, problems can arise when such silence is misinterpreted. Your *child* may assume that your silence means you do not really believe *he or she* is sick. There is no harm in maintaining a brave, stoic front, as long as you are careful to make sure your child feels your support.

As these fathers learned, the solution to this is for fathers to talk with their children, explaining that it is difficult for dads to watch as their children suffer. In trying to protect their YPWCs from their fears through silence, these dads found they may actually have been adding to the YPWCs' fears.

Communication

Maintaining open and honest communication may be the most important thing parents can do. Your family may be traditional, with all members living together under one roof, or a single-parent family, with the other parent having visitation rights. Whatever the living arrangement, you need to understand each other's role and be able to work together for the good of your child. Once you understand each other's feelings and reactions, you will be better able to focus your attention on the situation at hand. If you can pull together in the same direction, it will be easier to come to terms with the many issues ahead—medical, educational, and family. When faced with a child with CFIDS, even the most "in tune" couples find they disagree on more things than they once did. There are so many new issues to consider, from school attendance to which doctor to listen to. Simple things, such as whether your child should get dressed every day, can become areas of disagreement between the two of you. For this reason, it is important to discuss everything. We know how difficult this can be; it takes time and patience, something you have little of when parenting a YPWC. We mention this as something to work toward, in the hope that it will help to ease the burden for both of you.

Usually, by the time this illness strikes, you have already established standards for your children in terms of behavior, expectations, and discipline. Many of these decisions will now come into question. Issues such as television time restrictions and daily exercise expectations may no longer be applicable. You and your spouse must be able to talk with each other and be willing to change many established routines. Parents can become so bogged down with the little everyday issues that they miss the big picture; they attempt to correct the situation by controlling the child. In the past, setting limits and expectations could curb inappropriate behavior, and in trying to figure out how to help our now ill children, we return to the comfortable devices that always worked before. We believe that if we can take control, we can shape behavior. If we just make our children get up and go to school, they will not be sick. If we limit their TV time, they will not be cranky. If we get them to bed at a set time, they will sleep and be rested. If we just set the routine and force them to follow it, all their problems will be solved. Although it would be nice if life were that easy, it is not. As parents, bickering over the little things is sometimes easier than tackling the real issue. Unfortunately, this child is sick and not getting any better.

For one parent to accept the CFIDS diagnosis while the other continues to deny and question it is not unusual. Watching our children suffer with an illness that is not curable is difficult. We are raised to trust and believe in our doctors, and when they do not know what is wrong, it is natural to question whether anything is.

Whatever challenges you face, you must find time to talk to each other about the many problems that arise. Parents who can openly discuss their opinions about their child's care and come to some sort of consensus are going to be better able to be their child's advocates when addressing medical needs with the doctor and any school issues that arise. Such communication may be problematic for couples who are unaccustomed to sharing in this way. In most relationships, the role of advocate comes more naturally to one parent than to the other. How then do you come to a consensus? Some parental advocates believe it is easier simply to make the decisions rather than discussing matters beforehand with their partner, fearing that if the other parent does not agree with the plan, the conversation will become a battle. They may have avoided confrontations in the past by not asking for the other's opinions. Although this may work for some household decisions, the choices about how to help our YPWCs are usually better made together.

Set a time to talk alone. This may seem impossible to some parents, but it can be done. Engaging the children in an activity they enjoy may be enough, but you might need to arrange child care with a neighbor or a sitter to ensure an uninterrupted hour or two. We suggest first writing down the points for discussion that you believe are your priorities. Many issues may need to be addressed, so start with the most basic, such as educating your spouse about CFIDS. Often one parent will read a great deal on the topic and try to get the other to read the same resources to no avail. A tip some of us find useful is to mark or highlight important points we want our partners to read and ask that they at least read those. Spouses will often more readily accept information gained from a third party rather than that shared by a spouse. The more we try to talk with and to educate each other about our feelings and concerns, the more we feel empowered to help our YPWC. If both parents feel respected and a part of the decisions being made, they may feel less compelled to battle over the issues. Having your views appreciated can be very satisfying for both of you. Once you know that the other person will listen, you will feel more willing to share the responsibility of decision making.

Believing in Your Child

Doubts about a child's illness are more often expressed by one parent than the other. One parent is commonly full of doubts about the severity of the child's symptoms, the management of the illness, and the illness itself, and may be quite comfortable being vocal about them. The other parent may also have doubts but is less apt to express them, fearing the illness will become a self-fulfilling prophecy. This parent might believe that by questioning whether it is all in the child's mind, the illness might transform from something physical to something psychological. With one parent already having doubts and freely expressing them, the other may not want to add fuel to those thoughts. If he or she too has doubts, maybe something is being overlooked.

When your child is sick with something that doctors do not understand, such as CFIDS, you constantly question yourself. It is difficult to accept that your child can be so sick without the doctors being able to find the cause. As a parent, you may not know what could possibly be overlooked, but if something were, such as a psychological problem, then maybe more could be done for your child. When we begin to doubt our children's illness, it tears us up inside and may lead to the children doubting their own illness. It is hard enough for these kids to be sick all the time without the burden of doubt.

Unfortunately, doubts are a part of this illness for children. First, parents might wonder if the illness is real. Once the illness is accepted, they may question whether it is really severe or whether it is just a ploy to gain attention and sympathy. Finally, even if they believe in the illness and in their child's complaints, they have difficulty understanding how a child can be so incapacitated one minute and literally doing cartwheels the next. This can leave parents doubting how the child really feels—a very troublesome issue to resolve and one that, unfortunately, some parents never do. Many parents have noted that the child complains of feeling awful when they are around, but when friends or relatives come over, the child appears fine. One YPWC's mother had this insight on the topic:

> I think my child is more likely to fake feeling well than fake feeling sick. When she feels bad so much of the time, what would she have to gain by pretending to feel bad when she doesn't? She would never waste those precious moments of feeling OK by feigning symptoms. When she feels so bad all the time, I have seen her pretend to be fine so she won't have to answer questions or see others' concern. Sometimes it can help to make her feel a little more normal for a short time.

Nurturing Yourself and Your Relationship

Along with communication, couples need time away to rejuvenate so they can be the best caregivers possible. This can be difficult when having to attend to a child's needs for twenty-four hours a day, seven days a week, for months at a time. Several couples from a family support group had the following comments on the issue:

> We needed to find time alone as a couple. Parenting two children with CFIDS had become an all-consuming struggle, and we needed to put space between our relationship, and the one we each shared with the children. It was not easy to go out the first time. We felt so guilty leaving them. But you know, they survived and actually were better when we were gone. They needed the break as much as we did.
>
> This does not need to be a whole day away. It may be something as simple as a walk around the block or a half hour alone to just talk.

Some mothers and/or fathers have difficulty accepting the fact that they cannot do everything themselves. Learning to accept help from family or friends or to ask for help when it is needed is not always easy. Parenting a chronically ill child can be an overwhelming task. Caregivers must guard against becoming frustrated and depressed when they feel unable to manage.

Being a child's primary caregiver and advocate is a monumental task. Caregivers' days are filled with school work, driving children to and from school, doctor's visits, activities, and filling the YPWC's days when he or she is not feeling well enough for a normal routine. The younger your child and the more this illness consumes your life, the more important it will be to find time alone. A warm bath, exercise, and reading a good book are all quick escapes that we have used in our own homes. Anything that allows you to shift your focus from caregiving for a little while will help. Caregivers need time to rejuvenate to better cope with their responsibilities.

We all must take time to examine our children's roles in our family. The YPWC, although ill, still needs to feel an important part of the family. This can be accomplished with a little caring and flexibility in planning. If you have other children, their needs must also be addressed. Their roles in your family should not be diminished because one of their siblings is ill.

Good communication is essential to coping with this illness. When we, as mothers and fathers, understand how our biological roles in caregiving differ, we can better understand the dilemma each of us faces in dealing with this illness. Moms help children to feel safe and secure in their worlds, while Dads ensure that their children are prepared for the harsh realities of life outside the cozy cocoon of home.

Parents help their children grow and develop into young adults who are able to face the challenges of life beyond childhood. Learning to appreciate and accept the differences in parenting roles may help to create more harmony in your home. You can begin to accept the strengths and weaknesses of your parenting partner and become bound together in a renewed resolve to fight for what is best for your child.

Chapter 4

How to Be Your Child's #1 Advocate

Believe and trust in your child!
You know your child and the situation better than anyone.

HOW TO HAVE A GOOD RELATIONSHIP WITH YOUR CHILD'S DOCTOR

Everyone should have a good working relationship with his or her doctor. However, with an illness such as CFIDS, this relationship is critical. Some families are fortunate enough to have developed a trusting rapport with a doctor who knows them and their child. When this is the case and the child becomes ill, the doctor knows from past experience with this family that something is physically wrong. The doctor can then work with the family to try to find the answers.

However, what more commonly occurs is that the doctor who has always been there for you is suddenly unwilling to accept that your child has an illness which cannot be diagnosed definitively with lab tests. Unfortunately, nowadays, more doctors are being trained as diagnosticians than as clinicians. They learn all the intricacies of how to diagnose and treat illnesses. The parent mentions two or three symptoms, and the doctor has a plan formulated and tests ordered before the parent has even begun to scratch the surface of the problem at hand. Fewer and fewer doctors take the time to sit and listen to the patient because they believe lab tests will tell all there is to know.

Frequently, the parent has to educate the physician about this disease and provide information and documentation on CFIDS. You may want to furnish a journal or a chart of your child's symptoms to help your doctor understand the magnitude or severity of your YPWC's condition. This may be enough for your doctor to take notice, but if he or she still seems uninterested in your observations, it may be time to consider another doctor.

Finding a doctor who will really listen and try to understand what you are saying is, unfortunately, not an easy task. This can be even more difficult if your family has medical insurance through an HMO (Health Maintenance Organization) that has a limited number of doctors from which to choose. In that case, you may need to consider paying extra money to see a doctor outside of your HMO who will listen. If your family is having trouble finding a supportive medical advisor, have a heart-to-heart talk with your child; explain that although some doctors do not believe in CFIDS or do not know about it does *not* mean that CFIDS does not exist and that he or she is not sick.

As difficult as all this is, most parents have said that it was well worth the effort in the long run. CFIDS is an illness that does not go away overnight. Good medical care is essential. Trusting and having faith in your physician is critical. When you put your child's care into the hands of someone you believe in, you can trust that only necessary testing and treatments will be recommended. Sometimes all your doctor has to offer is support, understanding, and compassion. Simply feeling that you are not alone will be a tremendous help when struggling to cope with this situation. And for your child, compassionate support can be as vital an aspect of the healing process as medications.

Medical Records

It is quite common for your child to be seen by a number of doctors and specialists before the diagnosis of CFIDS is made. This can be a very frustrating time. You may feel lost, not knowing where to turn next. As you go from doctor to doctor, the list of referrals may grow; each physician knows another physician who can probably help you and your child. You begin to feel as if you are on a winding road where you can no longer see the beginning, and you keep hoping the end is just around the next bend. You will find it easy to lose your perspective amidst this sea of medical opinions.

One way to ease this confusion and regain your perspective is to ensure that your primary care physician receives a copy of each doctor's medical report. Most will send a copy to the doctor who referred you, but, if requested, they will also send it to any other physician you name. You should also request a copy of the report for your own records. Assuming your primary care physician is the one with whom you feel most comfortable conferring, you can periodically arrange an appointment to consult him or her on what is happening.

With an illness such as CFIDS, keeping copies of all your child's medical records is advisable. This includes reports of all lab tests and diagnostic procedures, as well as physician's reports. In most states, when patients request their physician to forward *all* their medical records to another physician, there are limits as to what can be sent. The law in many places is that forwarding physicians may forward *only* those records which have been generated under their care. They may *not* forward any records that they have received from any other physician or medical facility. Many parents have learned to bring along all copies of test results and procedures that their child has had whenever they see a new doctor. This saves time and money and minimizes your child's discomfort since tests are not unnecessarily repeated. It may also assist the doctor in making a diagnosis.

Finding a Support Person for Doctor's Visits

When possible, both parents should accompany the YPWC to doctor's appointments. This shows your child that both of you are searching for answers to his or her problem. It also helps your doctor get a clearer picture of the situation by hearing each parent's view of the symptoms. Sometimes this will not be an option, such as with conflicting work schedules or in single-parent families. However, we recommend that you bring along a support person who knows your child and the situation—a grandparent, relative, or family friend.

Going to one doctor's appointment after another can be over-whelming. In your efforts to communicate *all your* concerns to your physician, you may find it difficult to focus on the information the physician is attempting to share with you. To make the most of these visits, many of us bring along small, handheld tape recorders. By taping the appointment, you can refer back to points your doctor makes, check explanations, and have a record of the doctor's plans and ideas.

Misinterpreting what a person says or how a person feels is easy—tone of voice, attitude, and body language can cloud a person's perception of what is being said. Doctors are no exception. Having someone else to talk to or a tape to refer to can help clear up misconceptions or questions as to what actually transpired. When you have another person with you, you can talk afterward and compare notes and opinions of how the appointment went, which is especially helpful because two people often remember very different aspects of the same experience. For couples, sharing the doctor's findings and opinions following the appointment brings them closer together and helps them to feel united in their efforts to determine what ails their child.

A Trusting Relationship

YPWCs have special needs that require a doctor's support and acceptance. Your physician not only attends to your child's symptoms; he or she also is the one who writes letters to the school to ensure that your YPWC gets needed educational services—a limited schedule, a home tutor, or a waiver for physical education (see Appendix D for sample letters). Your doctor may also need to talk to school personnel about your child's condition. He or she may often play a key role in securing a good educational plan for your child by clarifying that the disability or health impairment exists. For all these reasons, as well as for your own comfort, you should have a doctor you can trust, one with whom you can work.

HOW TO BE YOUR CHILD'S ADVOCATE AT SCHOOL

Communication is the key to a workable school plan.

Approaching the School

You will find many suggestions throughout this book about how to devise a workable school plan. Your child may attend school only part of the day, or he or she may need to rest in the nurse's office to get through the day. Some children may need to use a tape recorder to assist in note taking or a calculator for math computation. Whatever the needs, it is up to you as the parent to see that your child is guaranteed and receives the services to which he or she is entitled.

Approach the school staff knowing that giving your child a good education is their top priority. However, remember that you have only one child's interests at heart; the school personnel are responsible for hundreds of children's interests, and the school's job is to provide each child with the best education possible. When meeting with the school staff, many parents find it helpful to convey an attitude of confidence in the school's ability to educate their child. This goes a long way toward building a positive relationship.

As easy as that sounds, you also have to be prepared at times to fight for what is best for your child. When your child is unable to tolerate physical education, you can get a medical excuse from your doctor to have your child exempted. You should encourage your child to be as active as possible so he or she will get some exercise and physical activity, but in doing so, you may create another problem with school staff. For example, one adolescent could not attend physical education class (which was the first period of the day) and still be able to get through the rest of the morning. However, she could tolerate cheerleading because she had a chance to rest after school, go to cheerleading and perform at her ability level, and then return home to rest/sleep. You may have to explain repeatedly to the school staff why your child cannot tolerate physical education during the day but can participate in certain physical activities outside of school—the reason being that rest can occur before, during, and immediately after the activity.

Maintaining Contact

Some days it seems that no one really understands. Your spouse may say you are being overprotective; teachers want assignments; and school personnel need more information from you. Hang in there; it is worth the effort. Keep talking to the teachers and other school personnel and explain what you need. Teachers are very busy with the students they have in their classes and may not see the value of preparing materials for home instruction for a child too ill to attend school. As your child's advocate, you must make your child a person in these teachers' eyes. They need a face to go with your child's name, and they need a personal interest in this individual child. One way to do this is to take your YPWC in for conferences. When the teachers see your child and hear what life with CFIDS is like from your child's perspective, they may gain not only insights but more interest in helping your child, who is fighting so hard to help himself or herself. Teachers may see your child as homebound and not realize how driven most YPWCs are. Your job as parents is to keep reminding these teachers that your homebound student has a face and a name, and he or she wants and needs each teacher's help. If you do not fight for an equal education for your child, no one else will.

When everything appears overwhelming, and, as a parent, even you are unsure of what your child can manage, you may not know where to turn. Parents who have had successful relationships with school staff have one element in common: COMMUNICATION! They did not make just one visit to the guidance counselor, but kept up an ongoing communication with all of their child's teachers. The following material presents some suggestions on how to be a successful communicator.

Arrange a meeting at the time of diagnosis with anyone on the school staff involved with your YPWC. The guidance counselor can help set up this meeting. Included should be the counselor, all your child's teachers, and the school nurse. Inviting the principal, or at least informing him or her of the outcome of the meeting, is also a wise idea in building bridges with the school. You can share with these people the symptoms your child is experiencing and then present what you and your child's physician recommend in terms of the school program. (See Appendix D for sample letters.)

Some parents have found it best not to try to educate the teachers on all the ins and outs of CFIDS. They concentrate on what their children are capable of doing instead of what they cannot do. By telling the school what the child "can do," you put a more positive spin on the situation. Your child's accomplishments may be as simple as taking a shower or eating independently; they could also include being able to walk unassisted to the mailbox and back. This helps to portray your child as a doer and not as an invalid. Parents have found that this can affect the teachers' perspectives and make them more receptive. Sharing some of the brochures and literature related to children with CFIDS has also been useful for some (see Appendix B—contact support groups for brochures). The best advice is to keep your information simple and relevant.

At the beginning of the school year, meet with all of your child's teachers, as was done at the time of diagnosis. You can share with them how things have been handled, what has and has not been helpful, and how your child is doing now. If special arrangements have been made for your child to attend an abbreviated school day, share this with the teachers. It is your responsibility, as well as the counselor's, to keep the teachers informed of what is going on, whether there are changes in your child's health, and what changes in school arrangements have been made. A positive, cooperative attitude goes a long way toward getting your child the services he or she needs and deserves.

Maintaining contact with the school staff throughout the year is essential. Some parents find that a bimonthly or quarterly note to teachers about their YPWC's condition can be very helpful, especially for those teachers with whom your child may be having trouble. The discussion can include how your YPWC is managing schoolwork. Teachers may not know how much difficulty your child is having with reading or computation if all they see is the completed assignment. They may have no idea of the effort that went into the assignment. Every time there is a major change in your child's condition, let the teachers know. Some parents have found that updating the nurse or guidance counselor on the YPWC's condition does not necessarily mean that all the teachers will also be informed. Informing everyone directly will help avoid misunderstandings. Encourage the teachers to call you if they have any questions or concerns.

At midterm and finals time, it is advisable to meet again with your child's teachers to ensure that any agreed-upon modifications in testing are made. Although your YPWC's educational plan may include the use of a calculator on all math tests, the teacher may not allow it on the final unless reminded of this accommodation.

Near the end of the school year (April to May), it is good to meet with the guidance counselor to start planning for the following year. Be aware that although there are no guarantees, requests may be put in your child's file for specific teachers and schedules. You can then touch base before the start of the year to make sure the schedule is suitable and to inform the school of your YPWC's condition. Some children who were very sick in June may be able to go full days for the first few weeks or months of school, and should do so, if possible. If this is the case, the most important extra classes (such as art or health) should be scheduled for the first marking period. If the counselor is aware that although your child is attending full-time this week, he or she may not be able to do so for long, plans can be made accordingly.

FURTHER CONSIDERATIONS

For children who suffer from a minor case of CFIDS, the previous accommodations and arrangements may suit their educational needs. However, if you have followed these suggestions and your child is still not functioning at a pre-illness level of achievement, you may wish to ask yourself these questions: Is my child the student he or she was before becoming ill? Is he or she happy about the way school is going now? Could my child benefit from modifications in homework requirements and teacher expectations? If you answered yes to any of these questions, then you may wish to fine-tune your advocacy efforts. You can request an individual education evaluation of your child to see if he or she qualifies for special educational services. (The decision to classify your child and some educational planning options are discussed briefly in Chapter 8.)

The following material includes suggestions for preparing yourself to meet with school personnel and the Committee on Special Education (CSE). Our experience has been that services for our special children are not always easy to obtain. Most parents who have been successful in getting special services for their child have fought hard. Hopefully, the tips that follow will assist you in your quest to get your child the best education possible.

If you have not already done so, start creating a "paper trail" of your school communications by documenting all your contacts. One easy way to do this is to use a spiral notebook and a pocket folder. Every time you talk to someone at the school, make a note of it in your notebook; remember to include the date, person's name, and the nature of the conversation. Keep copies of all correspondence, received and sent. This may include requests for assignments, updates on your child's health, and even the occasional thank-you notes written to teachers and others who have been helpful and supportive. Remembering to write notes of appreciation (and sending copies of them to the principal and the superintendent, etc.) will show your desire to work with the school personnel and not against them. We all like to be appreciated, but to be acknowledged to our superiors provides even greater recognition. People who like you will go out of their way to help you.

Meeting with the Committee on Special Education: How to Prepare

Before the Meeting

1. *Try to adopt an "I can" attitude.* Keeping a positive attitude about what you are doing and why can make a big difference.
2. *Become familiar with your child's past achievements* and have documentation to back up your claims. Secure copies of old report cards, teacher comments, and standardized test results. Keep these together in one place with current test results. It is not unusual for your child to test in the average range on standardized academic tests that show achievement and potential strengths/weaknesses.

   For example, parents attempting to obtain services for their son were told that the CSE did not feel the services were necessary because their child was maintaining his grade level standing. They were ready to deny him services based solely on their testing. No one took the time to check the records, which showed that he had been in the superior range in math performance, based on standardized test scores in elementary school. He had fallen from the ninety-eighth percentile to the thirty-sixth percentile in math in two years' time. Initially, only 2 percent of children his age taking the test performed better than he did. Eventually, 64 percent of the children his age taking the test performed better than he did. This is a significant drop that would not have been brought to the CSE's attention had the parents not secured the information themselves and presented it at the hearing for classification.

3. *Know the laws as they pertain to your child.* Have copies of the laws with you so that you can quote from them if necessary. The CSE may never have had a student who was classified under the "Other Health Impaired" classification, and may not know how CFIDS fits that criterion (see Chapter 8).

4. *Have a medical report from your child's physician* that explains why CFIDS is considered an "Other Health Impairment" and how it affects your child's "educational performance" (see Appendix D).

5. Although *you might see clearly why your child deserves certain services,* the school staff might not. The CSE is more accustomed to convincing a parent to allow services for the severely impaired child than it is to having a parent fight to get a child classified. They may not see a need to classify your child and believe they are already providing the needed services.

6. *Build a solid case for your child.* Try not to become discouraged. This is, of course, easier said than done. Keep in mind that your child has the right to achieve his or her pre-illness level. Be polite and persistent in your efforts to get services.

7. *Write an outline of what you plan to cover at the meeting.* Include topics, questions, and any other concerns you need addressed.

8. *Ask for a list of the people who will be at the meeting.* Knowing the names and titles ahead of time will help you prepare. Facing a room full of people when you were not expecting to can be overwhelming.

9. *Plan to take someone with you to the meeting.* This may be your spouse, a friend, or anyone who can be there to support you and your child if needed. You may even hire a professional advocate to be there on your behalf, if necessary. Decide who will be the primary spokesperson for your child. Devise a

signal with this support person so if one of you gets off the track or angry, the other can offer a reminder to stay focused (a gentle touch on the arm or a tap of the finger should suffice).

On the Day of the Meeting

1. *Dress appropriately.* When you look your best, it shows that you respect those at the meeting and that you take this time very seriously. Some parents find that dressing professionally puts them on a more equal footing with the staff.
2. *Be on time for the meeting.* Arriving a little early is better than being late.
3. *Bring a pad of paper and a pen to write notes.* During the meeting, jot down any suggestions and/or promises that the committee makes. It is very difficult to remember everything that is said without a record. You can even request permission to tape the meeting if you wish; it is your right to do so, but you need to request this beforehand.
4. *As people arrive for the meeting, stand, shake their hands, and introduce yourself,* if no one else does. People are more apt to listen to you if you first set a tone of mutual respect. This can be difficult if you have not had a good rapport up to this point. Setting a positive tone will help obtain the accommodations/ services your child needs.

During the Meeting

1. *Seat yourself so that you can maintain eye contact* with every-one present, especially the chairperson of the committee. Try to maintain an open body stance. Crossing your arms and legs can suggest "I am not listening to or agreeing with you."
2. *Speak when spoken to.* Try to listen to others, and do not interrupt when they are talking. This can be very difficult at times. If you wish to make a point, write it down so you do not forget. Make a request calmly and firmly to speak next. You may have to remind others that you gave them their turn to voice their opinions and now it is your turn.

3. *Stay calm.* Do not raise your voice or insult anyone. Try to be concise and not ramble. This is where good preparation comes into play. If you keep referring back to the notes that you came with, you can continually bring the meeting back to these points. The bottom line is this—the more you *know your rights,* and can *state them confidently,* the better chance you have of being successful in securing services for your child.

4. *If the meeting seems to be going nowhere* and you find yourself becoming lost and frustrated, you have the right to request that the meeting "be tabled." You may explain that you need time to gather more information on whatever topic you are in disagreement over. Even only a short break to leave the room to cool off will help you regain your composure. The fastest way to lose credibility is to lose your temper and start ranting and raving at everyone.

5. *If you think the meeting is going in a nonproductive direction,* try to key in on a few critical points: What is in the best interest of my child? What is the *least restrictive environment* within the confines of CFIDS? (Whether the child is in school or able to sit for any length of time are important considerations.) Restate the laws that you are asking the committee to address (refer to Chapter 8).

After the Meeting

Do not become discouraged if the meeting does not go as well as you had expected. Go home, regroup, and make a list of what you accomplished and what you want to do next. Being your child's advocate is like traveling a long, winding road. We who are traveling this road will stumble many times and often feel lost, but somehow we keep going. Some stretches are easier than others, and sometimes the way is smooth. Other times, we might hit a roadblock and have to go back to the beginning and start all over again.

Securing the best educational program for your child is only the beginning. Your role as your child's advocate does not end when "promised" certain services. As your child grows and changes teachers and schools, you will need to reacquaint yourself with new administrators and other school staff. Being prepared for possible pitfalls will make these changes easier in the long run. We all wish that we could just get the plan in place, sit back, and not worry. Unfortunately, that is rarely the case. There are always new people to explain your child's program to and people who have forgotten what accommodations have been made. As parents, each of us must be prepared to be our child's advocate—today, tomorrow, and throughout life.

Chapter 5

Helping Your YPWC
Develop Socially

Following medical treatment for CFIDS, one of the biggest challenges we as parents must confront is helping our YPWC with socialization. We have all spent nights grieving the loss of our child's friendships and the missed opportunities that our YPWCs face as a part of this insidious illness. We hear the parents of healthy teenagers complain that their children are never home due to all of their activities and social engagements, while we long for the rare invitation for our YPWC. The following are some YPWCs' comments about how CFIDS has affected their lives:

> When I haven't been to school for a while, I feel left out when I go. My best friend always understands. The other kids in my class, who used to be my friends, are like strangers. (seven-year-old girl)

> I am glad to get out to see people at school, even if it is only for one period. I wouldn't want to be home all the time. And about my friends? You mean the friends before CFIDS or now? (thirteen-year-old boy)

> How appropriate that I missed Senior Day. I was invisible during the four years I was there and never really belonged anyway. (eighteen-year-old girl)

These children—who want so much to belong, to fit in, to have their lives back—become the forgotten classmate, the unpredictable friend, and the lonely student. Without our help, they could easily fall off the social ladder altogether and miss out on this critical period of social development. It does not have to be that way.

Social activity is a major part of a child's and adolescent's existence. It helps children define who they are in their families and in their lives. As they grow, children move from the security of their family into a world that can be frightening and overwhelming. They attempt to find ways to fit into the world and become independent and self-reliant. They develop positive self-esteem through activities that help them feel competent and needed. As the years go by, the desire for social activity outside of the family increases.

Although young children with CFIDS certainly have social challenges, most of their interactions with people come through family activities. However, for adolescents, who are trying to break away from the family, the situation is more complex. They are struggling to develop their identity and some independence in their lives. Although they seek more support from people outside of the family, they still need their family's unconditional love and support, now more than ever. To continue to support your adolescents while encouraging them to venture out into the world is one of the many challenges of parenting. For children who are ill with CFIDS, this struggle can be phenomenal.

THE HEALTHY CHILD'S SOCIALIZATION

It may be easier to understand the changing social needs of YPWCs if you can understand what other children their age are experiencing. In elementary school, children normally interact with others in their class. Friendships develop easily between children who sit next to each other or who are in the same reading group. Children are trying out social skills in a very limited, safe setting. The classroom becomes like a family to the child, in that the children are all together, all day, every day. Young children tend to be very accepting of their peers. A child on crutches or in a wheelchair may actually gain socially because he or she is different; other students want to be this child's friend. This is very different from what children will experience in the teenage years.

At this age level, the majority of a child's social activities outside the school day revolve around the family. For the most part, children at this age are comfortable with their role in the family, and they acquire their feelings of self-worth from family relationships. This is safe for them. They begin the early stages of independence by forming friendships outside the family. Such friendships often exist for a relatively short period, and as these friendships dissolve, children will return to their family for emotional security. Having regained this security, they will gather strength to seek out new friendships.

As children reach the middle school or junior high years, their family is no longer the center of their social lives. Friendships outside of the family become the most important thing to them, and their friends begin to take up a great deal more of their time. They want more friends because, to them, popularity signifies acceptance.

While in the elementary years, a child is usually accepted unconditionally by peers; young adolescents are not nearly as supportive. Social activities, which have been part of family life up to this point, now take place at school. Classroom activities, school clubs, organizations, and athletic events are the center of students' social development. They seek group activities with their peers, such as athletic games and school dances, in place of family activities. Young adolescents need to be seen as a part of the group; their self-image is defined by what their friends think of them.

Young people do not want to be treated as children anymore. They try to act more adultlike and grown up, attempting to model many of the adult behaviors they see.

The middle school child needs the support of family and the contact and acceptance of friends. At this age, strong friendships may also begin to develop with other adults in the child's life. Adolescents often look to teachers for validation that they are indeed growing up and becoming young adults. They also look for acceptance from them. In elementary school, the teacher was a surrogate parent, so to speak, but in middle school, teachers are often mentors or friends to be admired and respected.

An adolescent will seek a balance between the family and the new social activities engaged in with peers. Supportive families make it much easier for a child to venture out into the world and test his or her independence, knowing that the safety of the family is always there when needed.

At this age, an interest in the opposite sex begins. Oftentimes simply talking to someone of another gender is a major hurdle to overcome. The sense of self that has been developing for several years is now challenged, as the budding teenager faces the insecurities of dealing with the opposite sex.

As adolescents enter high school, they move even closer to their friends and further away emotionally from their family. They rarely engage in family activities unless their friends are invited. Group activities are important, but what may be of more importance is having one or two close friends. Friends talk on the phone and write notes to each other to share all their feelings and problems. Adolescents value the acceptance of these few close friends more than that of their family.

While in the middle school years, children struggle to not be different; this is not as important as the teen matures. Teenagers tend to be more accepting of their friends' differences. If two teenagers develop a close relationship, they tend to remain best friends, supporting and encouraging each other through thick and thin.

By high school, being friends with members of the opposite sex is very important to adolescents. They need to feel accepted and liked. They usually begin to date, and quite often their relationships with boyfriends or girlfriends will come before their best friends. Teenagers often have difficulty balancing friendships and feelings during these years.

SOCIAL ISSUES FOR THE YPWC

The inability to interact with peers can be one of the most devastating long-term effects of CFIDS for your child. For this reason, you must help your child to become as involved with his or her peers as possible.

YPWCs who are able to maintain near-regular school attendance and to function at approximately the same level as children their own age will probably not suffer as much socially as one who is more restricted by this illness.

It is unusual for a child younger than ten to be diagnosed as having CFIDS. However, some children do develop symptoms during these years. At this early age, teachers model behavior for their students so it is important for them to understand the child's illness. If a teacher is understanding and accepting, then usually the students will be accepting. If the teacher labels this student as a malingerer, then the other students may do so as well. Teachers can be instrumental in shaping children's understanding of illnesses.

Children in the early grades suffer from a variety of aches and pains, such as stomachaches and headaches. Teachers often have difficulty discerning the normal aches and pains of healthy youngsters from the intense aches and pains of a child with CFIDS. (This is another reason to choose a supportive physician who can help teachers and others understand this illness.)

Adolescent YPWCs who attend school part-time may be labeled as "different" and stigmatized because of it. These children may be able to arrange a school schedule to have classes with some of their closest friends, allowing them to maintain their friendships and contacts. Even so, YPWCs cannot always engage in many extracurricular activities, which severely limits social contact with these classroom friends. Friends may not always understand why a YPWC cannot always keep commitments for plans made. They may also become impatient and intolerant of this sporadic schedule and stop making plans with the sick adolescent.

A homebound student faces the most difficult social situation. If your YPWC is unable to travel outside the home for school, then getting out of the house for social activities is problematic as well. Try to seek out a friend for your child in this situation—a cousin, a neighbor, or an old friend—anyone with whom your child feels comfortable and who will understand and tolerate the day-to-day fluctuations of this illness. Having this person stop by every week or so after school for a short visit is something your YPWC will truly begin to look forward to.

Sometimes your child will not be well enough to attend school for more than a portion of the school day. You may wish to try to have your child included in the social activities the school offers. Parents need to explain to teachers why their child cannot tolerate a full day of school. They also need to explain that, with rest before and after a field trip, their child can handle that activity. Schools can be very supportive if they understand the illness. Not every school will have supportive staff, but many do, and it is worthwhile talking to them to get your child involved in as many activities as he or she can manage, along with the academic program.

There are also many opportunities for socialization outside of school. Some YPWCs attend dance classes, library clubs, church youth groups, and other activities not affiliated with the school. On a Saturday afternoon, you can offer to drive your child and a friend to the mall or to a local movie theater. Just getting out of the house can be very rejuvenating for your child. Family activities should be encouraged, and unless too ill to attend, your child should participate. Even if it is tiring at Grandma's, there is usually a quiet place to lie down. Anticipate this need and bring along a drawing pad or quiet activities for when some "down" time is needed.

Other avenues of social contact are growing as pediatric CFIDS becomes more accepted. Several national support groups have information on this issue (see Appendix B). If there is no support group in your area, maybe your child would like to start one with others you know in this situation. A relatively new support network is on-line connection. Some services, such as America Online, have groups just for YPWCs that meet to talk via the electronic highway (see Appendix C for on-line resources).

Although these special youngsters may have a different introduction to the world of socialization, they need not be deprived of it. Parents of YPWCs have noted that although their children's contacts were limited, they have grown into strong, self-confident young adults who are more than ready to take on all the world has in store for them. They have remarkable coping skills, good communication skills, and a positive awareness of who they are. YPWCs, as they mature, gain in their own ways. They develop into the unique and competent individuals that we, as parents, feared would never be seen. (See Appendix G for Seventy-Five Tips for Coping with CFIDS in Children.)

Chapter 6

YPWCs and Parents Speak About Developmental Stages of Coping with CFIDS

In this chapter, YPWCs and their parents speak out about their experiences in coming to terms with CFIDS: Hope is their message. As YPWCs shared their stories, we were intrigued to note some amazing similarities and an overall sense of strength and hope in their accounts. We have woven their stories together for you into a tapestry of their common and unique experiences.

When YPWCs hear others' stories, many are astonished—and relieved—to learn how similar their thoughts and feelings are to those of other YPWCs, even when the other young people live in different communities or different countries. This feeling of shared experience is a powerful—even joyous—one, helping YPWCs accept more fully the reality of their illness—that they are not "weird" or "imagining things."

Although you can help your children by showing them how similar their experiences are to others with the same illness, it is also important to respect your child's individual experience with CFIDS. As we discussed in Chapter 1, CFIDS can present itself in mild, moderate, or severe forms, and with a variety of symptoms. Not all children are treated the same by their families and schools, and their individual personalities affect their ability to cope with their situation. All these differences add up to your child's own personal experience with the illness.

Note: Some of the YPWCs' quotes taken from stories mentioned in this chapter can be found at the Web site of Frank Albrecht, PhD, For Parents of Sick and Worn-Out Kids, located at: http://www.bluecrab.org/health/sickids/sickids.htm.

Because each child's experience with CFIDS is individual, the private tears and triumphs of these young people should be respected as uniquely their own. Nobody likes to be considered a "typical case" of anything. As parents, you should be aware that although another YPWC's account might seem to be "the same story" as your child's, it is not. Listening to your YPWC's individual experiences is one way you can really help your child deal with the illness. You can also help by ensuring that nobody tries to force your child into a mold. Even if some symptoms your child describes seem unusual or even unbelievable, remind others that doctors do not yet know everything there is to know about CFIDS. We all need to remember not to question the validity of what our YPWC is telling us, but to listen and to learn. In this chapter, we emphasize the importance of giving your child many opportunities to open up and talk.

In time, however, YPWCs need to move beyond just opening up and into a more active, coping frame of mind. Sharing experiences plays a role here too. Connecting with other YPWCs allows your children to learn from others' examples. As they chat with others, or read their stories, your children will not only feel more understood but will also be learning ways to manage their illness better. They learn both what can be helpful and what might cause a setback. If they are exposed to enough examples, they will also realize that the chances for significant improvement or recovery are good. These realizations can inspire the optimism and hope they need to carry on and move forward.

Twelve-year-old Jason finds the children's support group meetings very beneficial to his ability to cope with his illness:

> After a meeting I always feel drained and tired. But I also feel like I am not so alone. Knowing that those other kids are having the same problems that I am makes it easier for me. And also knowing that some of them have problems that I don't have, makes me feel lucky.

Although researchers are only just beginning to study coping in relation to pediatric CFIDS, they have noticed that the stages in this journey are very similar to the stages of coping and acceptance that occur with other illnesses and disabilities. The basic stages include some you may recognize such as "Denial," "Anger," and, in time,

"Acceptance." Other stages exist that are unique to CFIDS such as "Fighting the Diagnosis" and "Health Identity Confusion." No matter the name, these various stages are illustrated again and again by the words of these courageous youngsters and by the words of their families.

OBTAINING A DIAGNOSIS

Before your child was diagnosed, he or she inevitably experienced some changes in health that were worrying and confusing. Your child may have felt different even if the differences could not be put into words. Having many symptoms is difficult to understand, especially if your child had previously enjoyed good health. Even more stressful for your child is if he or she experienced a worsening of some familiar symptoms as well as the addition of new ones. For youngsters who became ill suddenly, recognizing this difference was probably easier, but no less painful, than for those whose symptoms came on gradually. The way that teachers, doctors, and you, as parents, reacted to your child's complaints about headaches, tiredness, and sore throats may be affecting how your child feels emotionally about being ill. We see how others' reactions affected one YPWC, Catherine Matheny, as told in her story, "I'm Wondering If My Time Will Come":

> My earliest recollection of feeling different because of CFS occurred in my last year of elementary school. I had been selected to be on safety patrol, which was a high honor indeed. I'd get up early every morning, strap on my bright orange belt, and take my assigned post, so proud of my responsibilities! Midway through the year, our faculty supervisor called me into his office and told me that I was missing too many days of school and he would have to take me off of the squad.
>
> I was crushed. This was the first time I recall feeling punished for not feeling well. This would be the first time I recall being criticized by my friends for not being around. This was the first time I felt that I could not rely on my body, or on myself. I felt humiliated, scared, angry, upset, but most of all, I felt confused. I was trying my hardest, but it wasn't good enough.

Sadly, Catherine's experience is all too common. Not only school personnel but also many families go through a period of disbelief regarding what their child is telling them. But, if you are reading this book after your child has been diagnosed, hopefully, that is in the past. Now is the time to "let bygones be bygones" and help your child move forward. When her child was finally diagnosed with CFIDS, one mother of a ten-year-old YPWC felt bad for the years she had forced her son to go to school with headaches, sore throats, and stomachaches. When she tried to apologize to her son, he told her, "I'm glad we didn't know what it was then and that we thought it was all allergies. I am glad to have had those years of 'feeling' like a normal kid with normal problems."

The stage of having symptoms but remaining undiagnosed may also create tremendous self-doubt in your YPWC. Without an accurate diagnosis, your child may be denied the proper medical care and may not be able to benefit from academic services for students with disabilities. In addition, without the correct diagnosis, children may fail to receive the social support they deserve. YPWCs may begin to question the symptoms and wonder if their problems are real or imaginary.

Receiving a diagnosis has a powerful influence on how children view their health. If doctors doubt that children are truly ill, then the children may also question the basis of the symptoms. Children often interpret others' skepticism as their own personal failure to cope with school and/or home demands.

Due to the widespread lack of acceptance for CFIDS, children may experience confusion, along with relief, when they receive the diagnosis. With other illnesses, the diagnosis will often help reassure the patient by identifying the problem and prescribing means to alleviate or cure the symptoms. This is generally not the case with CFIDS. The absence of abnormal diagnostic tests, however, does not justify ignoring these children's complaints. Following are the mixed feelings of several YPWCs about being diagnosed with CFIDS:

> I was elated. After all this time, and all the doctors and people who told me I was healthy and just not trying enough, or simply depressed, or suffering from some other not easily

diagnosed disease du jour it was exciting to have a CFS diagnosis. With all that I knew that it carried with it. . . . It was real. I was really sick. (Catherine—now age 24)

I felt relieved when I was finally diagnosed with CFS. I hated it when the doctors did not believe me. I was mad about going to the counselor. I was just happy to finally have a diagnosis. (Sam—age 10)

Part of me almost wanted something terrible to be wrong. Mainly to be able to say "See, I told you." . . . I also just wanted to *know* something. I think that I'm used to knowing things . . . it frustrates me when I don't. So, when I was told that I have chronic fatigue syndrome, I was somewhat relieved. At that time though, I didn't realize how so little is known about this disease. (Nichole—age 20)

"At last, a name for what I have," is a common sigh of relief expressed by many sufferers. Is it not ironic that for some, knowing that they have a real illness can occasionally make them feel better instead of worse? But for others, the diagnosis, although a relief in some ways, brings mixed blessings:

Strangely, I felt empty or "neutral," as I have come to call it. Nothing like the stereotypical reaction of denial, or bursting into tears, etc. Maybe because I knew that I had it anyway, I just hadn't had it officially confirmed. But even when the doctor was telling me about kids being ill for six years or more, I didn't feel much at all. Looking back, it was quite weird, I suppose. Maybe it was because it was too big a thing for me to acknowledge all at once, or maybe I was going through a kind of subconscious denial that I wasn't aware of on the surface. (Anna—age 17)

I felt that I was the only one. (Chris—age 11)

I was scared. My brother had CFIDS and I was afraid of getting as sick as he was. I was afraid I would have it forever. (Megan—age 8)

COMING TO TERMS WITH CFIDS

During the next stage, children attempt to come to terms with their illness and how it fits into their lives, which can be a long and slow process. First, they must learn what is a symptom of CFIDS and what is not. Even well-educated adults with CFIDS constantly wonder about this. When they get a headache, they ask themselves, "Is this CFIDS, or maybe just a virus? Is it a stress headache, or do I need new glasses?" Determining what is and is not a symptom of this illness is often difficult.

However, a number of informed YPWCs can outsmart adults in their knowledge of this complicated disorder! Lori, a sixteen-year-old YPWC, was one of those teens who took an intense interest in understanding her symptoms and learned more about her anatomy than most people care to know. She became obsessive and could describe her abdominal pain in a dozen ways, depending on where the pain was and how it felt. Her research in the study of anatomy was her way of coping with the illness, and this understanding allowed her a sense of control over her body.

There are also other YPWCs, who, depending on their level of abstract reasoning, may have a less sophisticated understanding of the human body than their parents and therefore find it difficult to grasp some of the complexities of CFIDS. They may not accept that overdoing it on Monday can cause a worsening of symptoms on Wednesday. They may absolutely refuse to become informed about their illness. The mother of a seventeen-year-old states:

> My daughter, Karen, literally threw the brochure about CFIDS across the room. It made me furious at first—since it had taken two long years to get the diagnosis and she was going to go to a special school all because I had struggled on her behalf. But then I realized she had little control over anything in her life anymore because of CFIDS. At least she could toss a brochure and feel she had some say about something.

Karen's reaction is normal among teenage children with CFIDS, and given how many doctors are baffled by this illness, it is not surprising. This type of resistance to accepting a diagnosis brings us to a priority topic with families who live with CFIDS: denial.

DENIAL

Denial is a very common human defense mechanism used by emotionally healthy people and is not, in itself, a sign of serious psychological problems. It is, in fact, a way of slowly coming to terms with something that might overwhelm a person if the truth were absorbed too fast. You need to be patient if your child shows signs of denial at the onset of illness and throughout its course. Denial is normal. It is cause for concern only when it interferes with the eventual adaptation to CFIDS that is needed to function properly in life. Such a judgment is difficult to make.

Denial is not an all-or-nothing stage. It can be there one moment and gone the next, only to return when you least expect it. Karen's mother, a PWC herself, states:

> Karen is at the stage when she admits she has CFIDS one day and denies it the next. This would be frustrating and even puzzling to me if I did not have CFIDS myself, and remember going through exactly this same process. The only difference is that I was thirty-six years old at the time. This helps me realize that Karen is not just a confused teenager. She's a person coming to terms with a challenging situation in exactly the same way as many more mature people do—in small steps and by taking two steps forward and one step back. As her parents, we have learned that we must be very patient as she struggles with this very tough task.

Some children become obsessive during this stage about engaging in normal activities they used to do. In an attempt to control something in their lives, they may become demanding over seemingly irrelevant things, as Andy's mother discovered:

> Andy became obsessive about shopping. While he used to enjoy getting out and going to the mall, now he demanded it. He insisted on going to the toy sections and then became irrational about buying certain toys or figures. At eleven years old, he behaved more like a two-year-old in the toy section. It wasn't until we sat down and discussed it that I realized there was little in his life that he could get excited about. When in

the toy aisle he felt like any other normal kid adding to his collection of figures. We worked with Andy to control his obsession, and gave him simple tasks to earn money to buy the treasured toys. Once he realized his obsession over shopping was really an attempt to regain a normal life in the face of CFIDS, he became more rational.

Andy's obsessions included denial of his illness coupled with anger over his inability to control his life. He was also facing the loss of normal activities and was grasping for what he still could manage, a day out shopping. As stated previously, denial may play a role in what is accepted as part of CFIDS and what is not. A child may be able to handle the incredible pain of stomachaches and sore throats better than they can accept the limitation in his or her activity level.

We do not know all the reasons why some kinds of symptoms seem acceptable to some YPWCs, whereas others do not. We do know, however, that all YPWCs grieve the loss of their healthy lives, and it is to that task we turn next.

LOSSES AND GRIEVING

Although helping your YPWC develop a coping frame of mind is essential, he or she must also learn to acknowledge losses as losses and to take the time—if given the opportunity—to grieve them. As one YPWC writes:

> When I look back over the past ten years, they are very painful memories. Instead of recalling football games and dances, dating and college, I see endless hours spent alone, feeling very ill. I see all the doctors and the diagnoses, all the treatments that I thought would be the cure. Watching my friends grow up and move on with their lives. This year, I'm watching my childhood friends graduate from college, and I'm wondering if my time will come. (Catherine—age 24)

CFIDS changes lives in very real and profound ways, and it is insensitive to minimize its effects. Although it is becoming more acceptable in our society for adults to disclose their pain and seek help for their losses, many young people do not feel this support and keep their pain deeply buried. It can be very stressful for YPWCs when their families and teachers constantly play the psychoanalyst. Despite this, you still need to be aware of the probability of your child's hidden sadness and worries, as illustrated by the words of this YPWC:

> Basically, I hardly see anyone. Prior to ME/CFIDS, I never really felt I fit in with my age group, and being ill has just emphasized that even more. I could be on another planet sometimes; my old friends' lives seem so totally irrelevant to mine. Mum worries about the isolation, but unlike a lot of YPWCs, I haven't found it that bad. . . . Because I find it hard to respect people who phone me once in a blue moon and whose only worries in life are who's going out with whom, I'm not going to jump at the chance to see them anymore. Mind you, that doesn't mean that it doesn't hurt, because it does. But the conversations we used to have just emphasized how different we were, and how separate our lives were, and so I don't really miss that contact. (Anna—age 17)

The difficulties in helping our children deal with these losses can be overcome in many ways. Seeking contact from outside the home, as suggested in Chapter 5 on socialization, will help them to feel less isolated. Encouraging them to write in a diary or journal, to engage in art activities or music, to care for pets, and to have pen pals are all time-honored methods to help YPWCs get in touch with their feelings.

The last comment we have on children's losses is the result of reading the words of the YPWCs we surveyed. The extent to which most of these youngsters grieve their loss of schooling is profound. Practically every YPWC stated, "I wish the teachers knew and believed how much I want to be in school!" This contrasts with the common misdiagnoses of "school avoidance or school phobia" and, as we have often stated, offers a compelling argument for working diligently to restore these children to as normal a school situation as possible.

DEPRESSION

YPWCs will feel their losses and grieve in a variety of ways. As parents, you must be aware of when the natural state of grieving turns to a more serious episode of depression.

Not all depression related to having CFIDS will be preventable, but the best protection you can offer your child is to keep the lines of communication open. Be available for and caring toward your child and always convey a nonjudgmental attitude. This will increase chances of your child opening up to you when he or she is feeling down. Getting your support and a different perspective may help prevent your child's depressive feelings. Even if depression does occur despite your best efforts, good communication in your family will likely lead your child to tell you when he or she is feeling depressed.

Adolescents cope with grief somewhat differently than adults do. Because of their tendency to think in black-and-white terms, they are inclined to view a negative event as a disaster, not just a temporary setback. This attitude predisposes them to feeling trapped or hopeless. Because they are less able to maintain a long-term perspective, matters that adults recognize as normal parts of teenage existence can overwhelm adolescents. If your YPWC is depressed, you, as the trusted adults in his or her life, must explain to him or her that no situation is hopeless and that there is always a way out. With teens, such feelings are especially common in relation to school and in matters of friendship. Tragically, much depression and even suicide in young people is related to being shamed or rejected. In the words of a father whose son was stricken with CFIDS this year:

> We had to go against the grain to help our son. While the people at the school and even our doctor were saying we should tell him if he didn't get better grades he would never graduate, we found ourselves reassuring Mike that a few Cs and even Ds were not the end of the world. It might take some time for us to get an educational plan in place that would enable him to succeed again. Making someone feel like a failure can lead to serious depression.

This father should know. As an adult with CFIDS, he became suicidal when he was asked to resign from his job because he was taking excessive sick leave.

We advise you, as parents of YPWCs, to take the time to talk frequently to your children, especially if they appear depressed. Tell them that you are always there for them and that they can talk to you about anything. If you establish open lines of communication, it will be easier to discuss negative feelings, which could lead to suicide without intervention. Ask them to promise to come to you if they ever feel so lost and alone that they are considering this option. Simply telling your child *repeatedly*, "I *love* you; you are the most important thing in my life," is important. But continuing on to say, "No matter what I am doing, always remember that you are my number one priority; I will always be there for you when you need me," may be all they need to hear to know how much you care.

When one mother of a YPWC, Samantha, was faced with her daughter's talk of suicide, she was speechless and did not know how to respond to her. Her first response was to tell her daughter how much she loved her and how much it would hurt her if she did anything to hurt herself. Then she and her daughter went through old photographs of wonderful times with loved ones. She told Samantha, "Every one of these pictures shows how much you mean to so many people. Think of what would happen if you were not in our lives." Samantha realized how lucky she was to have so many people who cared about her and loved her. She also realized how much she would hurt them, if she were to hurt herself. It helped her to put her life back into perspective.

If your child suffers from severe episodes of depression and has thoughts of suicide, treat these situations as emergencies. Talk to your child's doctor or counselor about a course of action.

ANGER

When you confront a person who is in denial, a common reaction is anger. This kind of anger can also erupt when YPWCs face evidence of the truth about themselves, such as realizing they misplaced their wallet for the third time in a month. Again, it is helpful to remember that the anger is a defensive reaction. Your YPWC is trying to protect himself or herself from having to face reality too quickly. Understanding and patience are called for in this situation.

As natural as it is, anger is still an overwhelming emotion for the families of YPWCs because anger can be so destructive to relationships. Even when parents have done everything right (and we have yet to meet such a family!), it is common for people with chronic illness to blame others, especially those who are supposed to be taking care of them. Try not to take the anger personally. Realize that this might be "CFIDS speaking" rather than your child.

Although uncomfortable being the apparent source of their child's angry outbursts, parents need to consider how draining and guilt-inducing this anger can be for their YPWC. After outbursts, YPWCs may feel as if they have alienated themselves from the very people whose support they need most. YPWCs may not be aware of the reason their anger makes them more anxious, but, underneath the rage, they may unconsciously feel profoundly insecure. Reading beneath the negative behavior can be a difficult task for parents and teachers. Although all young people need to learn to be respectful and nonabusive toward others, some extra compassion and patience is needed for these children who are dealing with one of life's most devastating illnesses.

Repeated angry outbursts may indicate the need for some outside counseling to help your child through this stage successfully. If the outbursts are mostly directed at you, then you may both be able to benefit from this. However, even if your child will not go to counseling, having a chance to unburden yourself of all your stress and worries may help you gain the perspective you need to deal with your child's anger. "No one can push my buttons better than my children can," one parent notes. "They seem to have been born knowing how to get the *reaction* from me that they are seeking."

However, remember that no matter what happened the day before, each day is a new beginning for you and your child. You may begin to feel overwhelmed and alienated from this angry teen, but remember—you are the adult, and your child needs you now more than ever. Start each day fresh with a forgiving attitude toward your child. Let your YPWC know that the slate has again been wiped clean. Sharing this loving, forgiving attitude on a daily basis may surprise your child, and you will both reap the benefits of your understanding and patience.

FIGHTING THE DIAGNOSIS

As discussed earlier, when your child receives the diagnosis, he or she may be very relieved to hear it. However, this does not mean that full acceptance of CFIDS has occurred. Having a name for their problems and accepting that this illness will possibly affect them for years is a lot for YPWCs, and their parents, to handle. It may even take years for your child to fully accept what this illness means. Some people with CFIDS never do.

Some YPWCs, as soon as they are diagnosed, will turn around and work vigorously to prove to themselves, and others, that the diagnosis is wrong. They may attempt to return to an old sport, stop taking their medications, and generally do everything they can to prove that they are fine. When you have spent months or even years, and possibly a lot of money, to find out what is wrong with your child, it can be frustrating to see this behavior. Also, since an increase in activities nearly always makes symptoms worse, you find yourselves having to watch your children get temporarily worse, not better. Although this is painful, it is helpful to remember that your child does not *"just have CFIDS."* Your child is also a developing person, testing the limits, proving he or she is normal, rejecting adult authority: these are all normal aspects of late childhood and adolescent development. CFIDS can complicate growing up if it interferes with these normal aspects of development.

We cannot stress enough how important it is not to disrupt the normal processes of growing up. You cannot jump in every time your teen decides that he or she can jog around the block. Hopefully, your child will learn from experience just how far to push the limits. Most parents opt not to force their YPWC to take medication if they choose not to, even if they can see how much it helps. Making a big scene over such matters nearly always aggravates the situation and harms your relationship with your child. You need to keep a trusting and open relationship. While children go through the normal stages of developing a separate identity, parents must allow them to experiment, make mistakes, and try new things. You will be surprised, however, when a couple of years down the road they "come back" to you. They may even criticize you for not "making" them listen when they were younger. And, as young adults, they may very well express their appreciation for all the support you showed them during those rocky adolescent years. The mother of twenty-year-old Brianna states:

> You couldn't ask for a more mature, considerate young woman. And she takes such good care of herself, cooking herself special meals, watching her sleep, organizing her time so she can continue her studies. We find it hard to believe that three years ago she was a lippy teen who once hid a doctor's requisition for a blood test from us.

However, not all adolescents—whether healthy or ill—go through a "rebellious" phase. In fact, research shows that most adolescents have a good relationship with their families and appreciate having some limits. Those YPWCs who, when healthy, were destined to have a smooth ride through their teens may be very cooperative with their parents and doctors.

As was discussed at length in Chapter 3, your child will cope much better with this illness if treated as much like a normal child as possible. YPWCs may actually fight the diagnosis less if they are allowed to feel that they are still the same people they were before the diagnosis. They need limits set, as all children do, and they need to feel a part of the family. You can do this by including them in family decisions, in choices about their health, in household chores, or having them participate in family outings. A mother of a fourteen-year-old YPWC shared the following:

> At night, I like to share some time with my son. Early in his illness, we began a ritual of backrubs at bedtime; however as he grew, they became less frequent. Needing to touch base with him more, I began offering them again. It relaxed him to be able to settle down to sleep. There is also something about physical contact that opens people up to talking. I always finish up with a kiss and a hug, and I LOVE YOU! It may only be a thirty-second rub, but it helps keep us connected nonetheless.

Lately he has taken to coming into my room near bedtime and sitting on the edge of my bed to talk. He freely chatters on about his day. No matter how tired I am, I listen. I know that these days will pass all too quickly, and that bonds of a lifetime are being built at my bedside. How do I know this? Because thirty years ago that was me at my parents' bedside chattering away, and feeling special, because they cared enough to listen to and be interested in me.

Watching your child begin to exhibit some of the normal behavior of a teenager can be quite difficult. As parents of YPWCs, our introduction to the turbulent teen years is much different from most. One trying task is determining what is normal teenage behavior and what is behavior related to CFIDS. The parents of another fourteen-year-old YPWC explain:

We were concerned that Nathan's intense interest in his new girlfriend was an attempt to escape coming to terms with his diagnosis. They literally talked on the phone for hours. This increased his fatigue. Then one day we had an accidental chat with some neighbors who have a healthy son of the same age. They were experiencing exactly the same problem! We laughed with relief when we realized that this was not CFIDS but typical teenage behavior. And, in that respect, it was a very healthy sign. Eventually we did set time limits on the phone so he would do his homework and to free up the phone for the rest of the family. We finally realized that having to set limits like this is a normal part of parenting a teen.

For many reasons, young people have different ways of coping with this illness. Some YPWCs just accept each day and seem to "roll with the punches," while others fight every symptom and problem with gusto. Just because your child is having a rough time does not mean you are a failure as a parent. Just because another family's YPWC is everybody's dream teenager does not mean that family is doing a better job than you are. Life is a lot more complicated than that.

REACHING OUT AND SHARING

Although we have stressed how important it is for YPWCs to have opportunities to share their experiences with others, we believe it is only fair to recognize that sharing can be a double-edged sword. Indeed, any time people open up and disclose their true feelings, they are taking a risk. If others do not really understand—and, to be fair, CFIDS is very difficult to understand—they may not believe what they hear. People often do not realize how much it hurts when they voice their disbelief. They also do not realize that this doubt may even make YPWCs question their own symptoms, as illustrated by the following:

> I'm usually positive that there is definitely something wrong going on in my body, but doubts do definitely creep in—many people in my own family don't believe I'm sick, don't believe CFS is real. They think it's all in my head . . . which hurts. But if they—my own family—can think that, then sometimes, yes, I begin doubting myself. It's a horrible feeling. Other people have said things too, some doctors included, but I can usually shrug off other people; it's hard and hurtful when it's your family. (Nichole—age 20)

Sharing can backfire if YPWCs feel they have earned a new label in place of CFIDS—"faker" or "liar." We asked eighteen-year-old Heidi, "Has anyone ever accused you of faking? Has that raised any doubts for you?" She stated:

> Yes, many times. School officials especially. People have made their feelings very clear. . . . The doubts I have are not because *I* don't think *I'm* sick; the doubts come from other people's disbelief. When people make it clear that they don't believe you, you automatically question whether or not you're really sick. Then you wake up the next day feeling really bad and wonder why you ever doubted yourself.

If your child's friends or relatives seem to feel this way, you may choose to try to educate these disbelievers about the illness. Grandparents, aunts, uncles, and others who do not visit your child on a regular basis may only see your child on an "up" day. By taking a little time to share the "quirks" of this illness with them, you may find they are far more accepting and understanding. At family parties, the parent of an eight-year-old YPWC uses comments such as "Boy is she going to feel sick as soon as we get in the car. I hate how she can push herself here, and look so normal, and crash so hard on the way home."

Being disbelieved is a common occurrence for those willing to share their diagnosis. Sometimes it is not the family or friends, but someone in the professional community who doubts. Joshua was ten years old and had recently been diagnosed by his family physician. His doctor knew virtually nothing about CFIDS and decided to send Joshua to a prestigious children's medical institute to talk to a specialist who claimed to have worked with children with CFIDS. In the parents' words, the following scenario unfolded:

> We were so excited to finally be meeting someone who could help Josh. As we shared his symptoms with the specialist, we began to feel that we knew more about this illness than this man who claimed to treat it did. After an extensive period of questioning, he asked to examine Josh alone, with two interns present. He said that the small examining room would not fit all of us, and would we mind waiting outside. When he was finished with his examination, he met with all of us in the room. He told us that Josh was in excellent health based on his physical examination. We tried to discuss some of the symptoms Josh had, but the doctor was not interested. He recommended that we insist Josh return to school, seek psychological counseling, and not worry about him.

In response to the parents' inquiry about his expertise in CFIDS, the doctor remarked that he had diagnosed one child, and that child had recovered. Josh's parents did not learn until later that during the private examination the doctor had tried to convince Joshua that it was all in his head, telling him he had to get on with life and stop pretending to be ill.

Even when others finally believe your child, they may not realize how much CFIDS affects your young person's life. The concept of an "invisible disability" is useful for explaining to your YPWC others' apparently cruel or indifferent behavior. It is easier to understand that others cannot really appreciate the effects of CFIDS when you realize that they truly cannot *see* most of the problems it causes.

IDENTITY FORMATION

Identity Confusion

One of the biggest differences between getting CFIDS when you are an adult and when you are a young person is that young people are still working on the developmental task of defining who they are—of forging an identity. The impact of the CFIDS experience on identity formation can be profound, as Catherine tells us:

> The loss of identity is the one thing that has been a constant negative for fifteen years. Also difficult has been the loss of trust in others who for years have disbelieved and doubted me. The final loss for me was the loss of my community—from the school, to church, to extracurricular activities. It was like my entire world disappeared.

This is an area in which you, as parents, teachers, and friends, can really help your YPWC. The first step in supporting identity formation is to minimize the extent to which the illness disrupts the normal processes of development. We have discussed this topic previously in several places, but it warrants mention here as well. This stage is critical for the adolescent attempting to develop a healthy self-image, as illustrated by Catherine's words. YPWCs who are labeled at this age as fakers or malingerers may suffer lifelong effects, as this label becomes burned into the core of their essence. For this reason, we believe getting an accurate diagnosis as early as possible is critical to the YPWCs normal identity formation.

The second step is to separate the YPWC from his or her disability. As we have already stated, you can remind your YPWC that although "you *have* CFIDS, you *are not* CFIDS." Continuing to treat your child as normally as possible will help in this situation, making your child feel like an integral part of the family and involving him or her in family activities as much as possible. If your words say, "You are not CFIDS," but your actions do not support this, your child will be confused and wonder where he or she fits into the family and into life.

A Continuous Sense of Self

The next aspect of identity formation is developing a continuous sense of self that links the past, present, and future. One common disclosure from YPWCs is that their memory of events when they first became ill is vague or even nonexistent. This can contribute to a deep sense of loss and also lead to gaps in general knowledge, as well as gaps in the kind of maturity that comes from experiencing the world. It is difficult to gain a solid sense of yourself when your life has been disrupted by an illness such as CFIDS. When others discuss past activities such as family or school festivities, YPWCs may feel sadness, anger, or resentment because they have little or no memory of such events. Here are practical ways that some YPWCs have compensated for these losses:

> My photo album has become one of my greatest treasures. It helped me keep connected to the past and the present and makes me feel I have a future. There are pictures of me when I was very active, pictures of me getting my CFIDS "chubbies," and pictures of me at the computer chatting with my new CFIDS pen pals. It's a mixed bag, but hey, this is my life; it's real, and it's connected. (Cassandra—age 17)

> As I was beginning to recover, my Mom helped me put together a resumé so I could apply for a volunteer job two hours a week. Just doing that made me see my life coming together. There was a gap in extracurricular activities in the ninth grade when I was too ill to do much, but seeing all my clubs and activities before that, and my prizes for poetry since then, made me feel like I really did have a meaningful life, after all. (Andrea—age 19)

Body Image

As parents of YPWCs, you have probably felt the pain of watching your children struggle with another aspect of identity formation—coming to terms with a body that has changed. Adapting to these changes takes time. Perhaps their bodies "do not work right," or maybe they have physical characteristics (e.g., rashes or weight gain) and assistive devices (e.g., crutches or wheelchairs) that can challenge any youngster. Nobody should underestimate the emotional pain that physical characteristics and assistive devices can cause youngsters and how much they dread being teased and humiliated. However, the world is full of examples of young adults who have truly come to terms with their "different" body images and who set shining examples to all of us about the strength of the human spirit.

You may be wondering how you can possibly make these struggles easier for your child. One way is to show your own acceptance of these changes. If it bothers you to have a wheelchair in the house, then it will be harder for your child to accept it too. Parents who continually comment on their children's weight will make them feel less comfortable with their bodies and solely responsible for the weight loss or gain. Although presenting a positive attitude is important for all teens, it is especially critical for the healthy development of our YPWCs who are struggling to accept the many changes they cannot control.

Aside from support within the family, another way to help YPWCs come to terms with this stage is to help them connect with other young people who have experienced similar changes. However, keep in mind that children and adolescents have a right to choose their own friends, and they may not want to go along with your plans to make connections for them.

Health Identity Confusion

Several researchers have noticed a complication in identity formation that they call "*health identity confusion*." Many YPWCs may have no memory of being completely well and are therefore not sure what health is and what illness is. Adults who became ill as children have stated that they are in good to excellent health while disclosing a significant number of current symptoms.

Children, in an attempt to convince doctors or teachers how ill they are, may even fabricate a sore ankle or a limp. Although this is not true "health identity confusion," it is an area that may cause concern for parents of children who are desperate to be believed. These children are not faking illness but are creating a symptom that can be seen, hoping to make it easier for others to believe them. In this situation, you may need to remind others that extra patience and understanding are necessary. Also helpful is for a YPWC's doctor to tell the youngster clearly, repeatedly, and in nonthreatening terms what the real diagnosis is and that CFIDS is *real*.

Another aspect of health identity confusion for your child may include cognitive problems associated with CFIDS. In Chapter 1, we discussed the descriptive terms that some YPWCs use for these changes such as "brain sludge" or "brain fog." But do not be fooled by the use of humor in relation to this topic; changes in mental functioning can be devastating to young people, and it is vital for your child to realize that these thinking problems "do not make you stupid."

Younger children, who learn at such a rapid pace, have not yet become aware of their learning strengths and weaknesses, making it almost impossible for them to judge the cognitive problems they may be experiencing. It may be easier for teens to recognize these changes and to discuss them with you. All children, however, will be affected by the attitude you take and by the expectations you hold. Actions speak louder than words. So, instead of saying, "I'll figure it out for you," when they struggle to calculate the cost of a purchase, wait patiently while they work it out, even if they have to use a calculator to do it. Not only does this help your child to solidify the skills needed, but it also conveys the message, "I think you are smart enough to do this."

A Future Identity

Developing a future identity is one of life's challenges that the older YPWC must face. These developing young adults cannot predict whether they will fully recover or what limitations, if any, they will have. As YPWCs are planning their futures, possibly applying to colleges, they may wonder if they will ever have a job, go to college, get married, raise a family—in effect, have the so-called "normal" life.

Parents and doctors may feel powerless to help the young person make plans for the future because they cannot predict the course of the illness either. Anything that is unpredictable is especially stressful. It is impossible to make CFIDS completely predictable, although learning as much as you can about the illness may help somewhat. More realistically, YPWCs need to learn how to deal more productively with unpredictability. The first step is to acknowledge how hard it is to live without plans. The second step is to celebrate the richer, more connected life that comes with "living for the moment" and "going with the flow." In a YPWC's words:

> I live day to day, and if there is something I want to do, I try to do it. With an uncertain future, this is the best way for me to live. That way I don't have my heart set on something only to be disappointed if I can't do it. (Heidi—age 18)

You can help your YPWC develop a future identity by moving away from rigid, black-and-white thinking about life. Helping your child to see that others have survived these difficult years, and have triumphed, is helpful. Your child does not have to be 100 percent recovered to reap the benefits of a normal life, hence the appearance of "health identity confusion" as discussed earlier. Some young adults will consider themselves fully or significantly recovered and in a state of good to excellent health, but still report having a number of symptoms related to CFIDS. These young adults, although unable to accurately determine their health status, are still managing to function and carry on completely normal and productive lives.

In a recent long-term study of YPWCs (currently being submitted for publication), 80 percent showed an overall positive outcome of their illness fifteen years after the onset of symptoms, while only 20 percent remained ill with significant health effects. For this reason, there is great hope for our children; whether or not their symptoms completely resolve, they can move on to have productive normal lives.

As adolescents struggle with these issues of their future and the uncertainty it brings, their parents cannot remove all their pain. The experiences of other YPWCs can help, such as those of Rebecca Moore, an advocate for all YPWCs:

I need to "send a note" to all of the younger YPWCs out there who feel trapped in that same bizarre world of an adolescent with CFIDS: it truly turned out all right for me! I'm no longer painfully shy, I smile more often than most folks I know, and I actually figured out how to do well in science class. My friends still are almost always either older or younger than I, but that is becoming an asset. I now know what my career goal is, and am confident that I'll achieve it by the time I have grandchildren. When I look back at the past four years, I see numerous times when God has worked in my life through people . . . guiding angels, if you will. Though I'll admit to having many fears about my future, and am feeling more frustration with my current limitations than I'd wish for, I am glad about who I am after my four years with CFIDS . . . and I think it's safe to assume that the next four years will be anything but dull.

ACCEPTANCE

The final stage of coping with CFIDS for YPWCs involves accepting that, for today, CFIDS is a part of their lives. At this point, YPWCs have grieved the loss of their previous health status and have stopped denying that their symptoms *may be* chronic. These young people no longer dwell on their previous academic abilities or activities, but have moved on to a life in which the limitations of CFIDS have become accepted:

The most important thing I've had to change to cope is my attitude. I've had to become a laid-back person. I have to weigh my priorities and consider my energy levels before I decide what I can handle, and if I can't handle something that day, I have to accept it. (Heidi—age 18)

This stage varies for different people. It does not mean that these young people have given up on their hopes and dreams. Acceptance is an individual phase that each person must go through. Research on coping with CFIDS in children has shown that YPWCs will try out many different coping methods in order to come to terms with their illness. They eventually will find a method that fits their individual needs and also those of their families. For some children, it may be smiling and being quiet about how they feel; for others, it will include overdoing it and paying the price later. Still others may choose to come to terms with this stage by extreme limit setting or overstructuring of their activities. No matter what style is chosen all are acceptable ways to come to terms with this illness, as long as the method "works" for them and for their families. Although their coping styles may differ, these children all hope for the same things: a world without CFIDS and a full recovery.

At this stage of acceptance, a YPWC no longer feels a need to completely hide the illness, nor a compelling need to share it with everyone. A more balanced view exists at this point, of when, where, how, why, and with whom to share information. Children also see their lives in a more balanced way. They can see the positive and negative aspects of their lives before CFIDS, as well as now. The unexpected benefits of having CFIDS are recognized; this may include a new appreciation for the abilities and interests they have developed due to CFIDS. YPWCs are more likely to appreciate the value of family support and strong friendships.

Along with this positive shift in perspective, YPWCs may develop a lively sense of humor. At support groups, you can hear them begin to tolerate some teasing about the illness as they share funny stories about their "fuzzy thinking" or about getting lost on the way to a familiar place. Teens may wear shirts with slogans such as "I used up all my sick days so I'm calling in Dead!"; the stressed-out stick figure that screams, "I can't take it anymore!"; or the Snoopy baseball cap with the sleeping snoopy, which one boy called his CFS hat. They may joke about creative ways they spent their time when hospitalized, such as the sisters who were admitted for IV treatments and found laughter in rides in the hallways of the hospital on their IV poles. Seeing them interact with their parents and each other in this lighthearted manner is heartwarming. Maturity, humor, perspective, and, above all, strength are the features that characterize so many of these courageous youngsters who have come to terms with CFIDS. Listen to the words of Jennifer as she shares her acceptance with the world:

If CFIDS makes you realize anything, it is that life is what you make of it. You can make it difficult or easy. With any illness, life changes and is more complex, but you can make it easier by letting go of the fact that you've been cheated out of what life you wanted to have. Think of why you were given this path of life. Maybe you will find something you've been looking for on the CFIDS path, as opposed to the path of a normal young person. Think about what you wanted your life to be about if you were not sick. Then think about what the CFIDS path of life has already given you. Would you have ever had time to literally stop and smell the roses, enjoy the chirping of a bird, or find out who you really are? You are a wonderful person, but would you have ever noticed? You were a smart and determined person before, but you have to realize that you are still that same person.

EDUCATIONAL ISSUES SURROUNDING CFIDS

Chapter 7

Deciding How Much
Your Child Can Do

HOW MANY HOURS OF SCHOOL
CAN YOUR YPWC MANAGE?

Of the many issues you will deal with in the course of this illness, one of the most difficult is how to organize your child's school day. No objective test or examination exists that will allow you to accurately estimate the amount of activity possible for your YPWC. The amount of quality time that children spend in school will have a profound effect on their entire adult lives, and you can help your child be more successful in school by learning some tips on "educational management."

To estimate just how long your child can be in school, you must consider several factors. Evaluating these factors is much easier if you have an open and honest relationship with your doctor. In fact, you cannot adequately evaluate your child's overall activity level without this. The goals of educational management are to keep your child at grade level and to allow as much socialization as possible.

Your first priority is to stress the importance of education. If your child was successful in school prior to developing CFIDS, this will not be difficult. However, children who did poorly prior to becoming ill will need help developing new habits and routines. Healthy children usually have time for school, extracurricular activities, homework, social activities, meals, and, unfortunately, television. For your child with CFIDS, the normal twelve to fourteen hours of available activity time will likely become two to ten hours. Obviously, the schedule that your child or adolescent followed before becoming ill will have to change. The trick is to fit productive learning time into this shortened day.

Consistency is the key when you are trying to decide on the amount of time in school that your child can tolerate, especially on a regular, daily basis. CFIDS is an illness of relapses and rebounds. The severity of the relapses may fluctuate from day to day and week to week and are often set off by increased exertion, physical activity, and even stress. It is quite common before diagnosis for YPWCs to attend school for a full day and then miss the next two to recover from the exertion. This leads to chaotic attendance, which further disrupts their education. CFIDS is also somewhat unpredictable. Although symptoms may worsen after exertion, it is not always possible to predict how someone will be feeling days or weeks in advance. So when you develop a schedule for school, it is critical to allow for flexibility.

A healthy school child will have twelve hours of inactivity (sleep, rest, or TV) and twelve hours of activity (school, study, play, sports, shopping, etc.) each day. For a YPWC with mild to moderate CFIDS, the activity range is generally sixteen hours of inactivity to eight hours of activity. It is important to note that the active hours do not have to be all at once. Even with frequent rest periods, this child would have a total of eight hours of activity in one day. A child with more severe CFIDS will probably have an activity range of twenty-one hours of inactivity to three hours of activity. Obviously, a YPWC with so few hours of total activity would not be successful attending school on a full-time basis.

No matter how many hours of activity are possible, help your child commit most of those hours to education. The formula we have found successful is three-fourths of activity time for education and one-fourth for social activities. If your YPWC is able to be consistently active for six hours a day, then committing four to five hours a day to education is reasonable. Remember that preparing to go to school, traveling to and from the building, attending classes/home tutoring, and homework all count as educational activity.

Another way to determine how many hours are appropriate for your YPWC to spend in school is what we call "the mall test." For many YPWCs, the mall is not particularly pleasant because of the loud noises, fluorescent lights, bustling activity, and crowds, but this is just what they encounter in the hallways at school. In reality, the mall is not as demanding as school. Although the physical stressors may be the same, walking the mall is a much more passive activity than going to school. Being in a classroom requires attentiveness and concentration, both of which create stress and drain energy. The mall test provides an easy way to gauge how many hours of consistent activity your child can tolerate in one day.

The test is very simple. On several given days, you can take your YPWC to the mall with a friend, beginning at around ten in the morning. If possible, the travel distance to the mall should be about the same as the travel distance would be to school. Your child does not have to be overly active. While you are reading a good book, your YPWC can wander slowly from store to store, resting in between on the benches that usually line the corridors. The mall test is not finished when your child first becomes tired. YPWCs usually will feel tired during this type of activity, and they should take time to rest. Do not leave the mall until your YPWC really can do no more, even after an adequate rest period. Use good sense here. Do not stay until the flulike malaise or exhaustion becomes severe, but do not leave at the first hint of fatigue either.

Your YPWC will probably require rest the following day, so you will know that the amount of time spent at the mall would be too much for a typical day at school. But through trial and error, allowing for good days and bad, you and your YPWC should be able to determine how many hours of "up time" or educational activity is possible. Once you know this, you can begin to plan for school.

Many parents and YPWCs are afraid to be seen in a public place such as the mall. This fear of getting "caught" can be extremely limiting and can prevent YPWCs from even a small amount of out-of-the-house activity. Both of you may fear that people will wonder how your YPWC is able to tolerate going to the mall, yet too sick to attend school full-time. Will whatever fragments of belief the school staff may have had in your YPWC dissolve into complete disbelief?

One way you can handle this is to enlist the help of your child's primary care physician. The physician should encourage increased activity within the bounds of common sense. If you discuss your plan to do the "mall test" with the physician, then it can be "approved" and not result in a surprise. The activity can be labeled "physical therapy" or "exercise"—not just goofing off. One drawback to the mall test is the expense, but this side effect can be avoided by going to the mall without money.

SCHEDULING YOUR YPWC'S DAYTIME HOURS

Once you determine how much activity your child can handle on a consistent and regular basis, you are better able to judge the length of your child's school day. If the mall test shows that six hours of activity can be tolerated, then four and one-half hours dedicated to education each day is a reasonable starting point. Courses can be scheduled for as much of this time as your child can tolerate, and tutoring can make up for the missed courses. Remember that educational time includes travel to school and homework, as well as time spent in classes and tutoring.

The most important courses to concentrate on are English, math, science, and social studies, but it is not always possible to schedule these courses together. If your YPWC can tolerate more than a few hours at school, you might want to separate two core courses with art or music, courses that usually cannot be made up through home tutoring.

One way to increase the amount of time your YPWC is able to stay in school is to schedule a longer rest period between classes. Some parents will bring their child home to rest during this time, while other YPWCs choose to stay in school and go to a quiet, secluded room to rest or sleep on a cot. If the nurse is supportive, that office may be the best place. Just by adding this simple measure, some YPWCs have been able to double the amount of time they are able to attend school, thereby avoiding home tutoring completely.

The following are five different school plans that have worked for other YPWCs. Your doctor and the staff at your child's school should help you to chart what course will be most successful. The success of these plans will be determined by the willingness of the school staff to work with you toward your YPWC's educational plan. These plans are not written as any legal guides, but were devised by schools and families working to find suitable alternatives to the normal school day:

1. *Complete home tutoring:* This option is necessary during relapses for YPWCs with severe illness. With complete home

tutoring, the core subjects are covered during the best time of your YPWC's day, often early or midafternoon. Tailor the length of these sessions to fit your YPWC's ability to remain alert and focused on academics.

2. *One or two classes per day:* In this option, the YPWC can consistently attend school for one or two important classes. This option is always preferable to complete home tutoring if your child can handle one or two hours out of the house. Just the act of getting dressed and going to school is therapeutic. Even a few hours of school will help your YPWC maintain social contact and attend school activities. With this option, your YPWC will require home tutoring for the subjects that cannot be taken at school.

3. *Half day of school:* In this option, the YPWC is consistently able to attend school for three or four hours and go to classes that are grouped during these hours. There should be no gym requirement. Special accommodations need to be made for transportation.

4. *Full day without gym:* With this option, YPWCs are able to attend school for all their regular classes, but do not take gym. If study halls or elective classes are scheduled at the beginning or end of the day, see if your child can skip them to allow more energy at home for homework. This option is used when the YPWC is clearly improving.

5. *Full day with gym:* YPWCs do not have to be completely free of symptoms for this option. However, they should have sufficient energy to complete all homework assignments consistently. Usually when this option is possible, full recovery will take place.

Good educational management is an important part of the ongoing care of the child or adolescent with CFIDS because it helps to minimize the amount of disruption that is caused by this illness. This includes determining the activity tolerance of the YPWC and tailoring the educational needs to this tolerance. The majority of YPWCs will be able to maintain grade level with an appropriate approach, and continue with higher education, an essential factor regardless of whether the illness resolves or not.

Chapter 8

Discussing Some of Your Child's Educational Options

Now that you have determined how much school your child can tolerate, it is time to look more closely at how the school staff can help you by addressing your child's special academic needs. Working toward securing the best educational program for your YPWC can be an emotion-filled task. It can also be very rewarding. In this chapter, you will read about some of your YPWC's educational options in the United States such as Section 504 of the Rehabilitation Act of 1973 and the Individuals with Disabilities Education Act (IDEA). Which option the school staff recommend will probably depend upon the extent of your child's educational needs and the amount of school your YPWC is able to attend. It is not our intent to instruct you on all of the ins and outs of these options. We hope to enlighten you with some choices and guide you in your search for information on obtaining the educational services to which your YPWC is entitled.

When your children get the flu and miss school for more than a few days, you probably respond by staying in contact with their teachers and getting their schoolwork, and you work with your children at home to try to keep them caught up with their classmates. Probably all of us started out this way with our YPWCs. When the staff at school are being supportive and are assisting you

---

Note: At the time of this writing, the provisions of the IDEA 1997 Reauthorization are going into effect. Currently, not all of the regulations are in effect and the states are examining them to incorporate any changes into their programs. All of the information in this chapter is accurate for your child now and under the 1997 reauthorization. Several additions, including components to the IEP, have been added. For more information on these additions, contact your local school district, state Education Department, or NICHCY (see Appendix E for addresses).

in keeping your child up to date with assignments, you may wonder why you should do anything else. Many of us were in the same situation and did not request any additional services for the first year or two. One of the authors had children who were sick in the 1980s when no one knew what this illness was or how long it would last. She knew nothing of the effects that this illness had on her children's ability to think and to function in the classroom. They thought the condition would just go away. Parents may have a variety of reasons for choosing not to have their child evaluated for special education services, and this is the first issue we will address in your educational program choices—doing nothing more than keeping in contact with the school.

WORKING WITH THE STAFF
ON A DAY-TO-DAY BASIS

Some parents are very reluctant to request special education services for their children. Parents sometimes worry that it will stigmatize their children in the eyes of friends and teachers. These parents may also have difficulty accepting that their children are really in need of additional services. In some districts, the school staff may be extremely helpful and supportive in providing the necessary accommodations to allow these children to achieve without the need for a specialized program.

Sometimes YPWCs can function quite well and reach their potential without being formally classified. This may be appropriate if your child has a mild case of CFIDS and is able to maintain nearly full attendance at school. The children mentioned previously who were sick in the 1980s were excellent students before they became ill. They managed to remain good students and graduated in the top ten of their class. The school system's personnel were willing to provide home tutors when the girls could not attend school, accept the doctor's request for no physical education classes, and allow the girls to rest as needed in the nurse's office. Their teachers were willing to go the extra mile to keep these girls caught up with their schoolwork. Be aware, however, that these are rather elaborate accommodations for a school system to provide without first doing an educational evaluation and at least setting up a 504 plan.

You may wonder why you should consider formalizing any alternative educational plan if you have a cooperative school such as the aforementioned one. If CFIDS were an illness from which your child would recover fully in two to six weeks, as is the case with many illnesses, then this would be a very adequate approach. In our experience with CFIDS, this is not the case. Although some YPWCs improve over the course of the year, few are well enough to function at their pre-illness level of activity on a regular basis.

Acting as your child's advocate can be an empowering experience. You are in the best position to offer information about what your child is capable of doing in regard to problems with CFIDS. Most school officials will not see the fluctuations in energy levels and cognitive abilities. They may not understand that walking from one end of the building to the other may bring on debilitating fatigue. Your child's teacher cannot see the mental confusion that your YPWC may suffer, or the pounding headaches your child may get when trying to listen to a lesson. The educators may not consider these problems when setting up an academic plan. As parents, you can help them to recognize the many challenges that your YPWC faces every day.

Hopefully, the people in your school district are willing to work with you. Such districts do exist and should be commended. However, you need to realize that without a more formal educational plan, the philosophy and procedures used to handle cases such as your child's can change at any time. This could happen if a new principal is hired at your child's school or when your child moves from one building to another, such as from elementary school to the middle school, or even changes districts. You may have found in the past that your child's principal was willing to accept CFIDS and ensured that your child received all the needed assistance. When a new principal takes over, you may find that the support and understanding you had received is no longer there. The new principal may question the CFIDS diagnosis and not be as willing to supply your child with the services that had been provided in the past. This person may believe that school phobia is the problem and that the solution is for your child to attend school on a regular basis.

As unfortunate as it is, this situation does exist. If your child has not been previously regarded as a 504 plan student, nor been determined to qualify for Special Education Services under the Individuals with Disabilities Education Act (IDEA), you will find yourself back at "square one." Rather than spending your time ensuring your child's educational needs are met, you will be seeking ways to convince this new principal that CFIDS is a real physical illness and not a psychological problem.

BECOME AWARE OF LAWS PERTAINING TO EDUCATION

Good communication with the staff at school is essential to your advocacy efforts. Hopefully, you have begun to build a positive rapport with the teachers and staff. This should ensure that your child receives all the possible benefits the school program has to offer. However, it is not always so. The school personnel you are working with may not be aware of how certain educational laws pertain to your child's condition. They also may not be aware of physical and/or cognitive problems that affect your child's educational performance.

Family Education Rights and Privacy Act (FERPA)

At this point, it may be helpful for you to become familiar with some of the laws that pertain to YPWCs and their education. The first of these federal laws is the Family Education Rights and Privacy Act—FERPA (20 U.S.C.A., Section 1232g, 1990)—also known as the Buckley Amendment. FERPA gives parents the right to "inspect and review the education records of their children." It also states that parents have the right to:

> challenge the content of such student's education records, in order to insure that the records are not inaccurate, misleading, or otherwise in violation of the privacy or other rights of students, and to provide an opportunity for the correction or deletion of any such inaccurate, misleading, or otherwise inappropriate data contained therein . . . (20 U.S.C.A., Section 1232g, 1990)

You may wonder why it is advisable to become familiar with your child's education records. Usually they contain only the objective information they should, such as old report cards and test scores. However, in some instances, parents have found unsubstantiated opinions, such as "He is a hypochondriac," which should not be a part of the record. Another reason to review the file is to become familiar with your YPWC's academic accomplishments. As discussed in Chapter 4, your child may have excelled in elementary school and had standardized test scores well above the average range. Suddenly, after the onset of CFIDS, you see a decline in test scores and achievements. This information can be useful in convincing the school of your child's need for services. The school staff may not notice the difference in achievement level and test scores if no one examines the past records carefully.

Rehabilitation Act of 1973—Section 504

Section 504 of the Rehabilitation Act of 1973 is not an education law but rather a civil rights law that prohibits discrimination against persons with a disability in any program receiving federal financial assistance. This includes public and private schools that receive federal financial assistance even if only for transportation or food service.

The act defines a person with a disability as anyone who:

1. has a mental or physical impairment which substantially limits one or more major life activities (such as caring for one's self, performing manual tasks, walking, seeing, hearing, speaking, breathing, learning, and working);
2. has a record of such an impairment; or
3. is regarded as having such an impairment. (29 U.S.C.A., Section 706 [8], 1997)

You may be asking yourself, "So, how does my child fit this definition of disabled under Section 504?" In our opinion, the words "substantially limits" in the first part of the definition are the key words to address. This does not mean that your child's physical condition makes it impossible to do certain things, but that he or she is "substantially limited" in this ability. For example, a normal child can walk around all day without breaks and not have any ill effects from such exertion. Most children with CFIDS are at least restricted in their ability to move around, as compared to healthy children, and may be unable to walk for more than a few minutes without a break because their stamina is affected. They may be unable to sit at a desk for the five to six hours that is required in a normal school day. They may have difficulty learning, concentrating, and writing. If they are limited in their ability to function at the level of their peers, then they are limited in one or more major life activities as listed in the definition. Practically all YPWCs are affected in at least one area, hence qualifying them for services. If you are reading this book, your child is most likely one of these children.

Included in the U.S. Department of Regulations guidelines for section 504 is the requirement that schools "establish standards and procedures for the evaluation and placement of persons who, because of a handicap, need or are believed to need special education or related services" (34 C.F.R., Section 104.35 [b], 1997). It also states that disabled students be provided with a free appropriate public education—FAPE (Section 104.33). School districts are thus required to identify, evaluate, and provide appropriate services for any student who is eligible. The school must "meet individual educational needs of handicapped persons as adequately as the needs of non-handicapped persons are met . . . " (Section 104.33 [b]).

If your child is identified as being able to benefit from a 504 plan, then the next step is to design a plan to meet your child's needs. Many of you may be concerned that if you allow your child to be serviced under the 504 plan, he or she will no longer be with peers in the regular education classroom. You may be comforted to know that the school must provide your child's education and needed services in the least restrictive environment (LRE) possible. As stated in Section 504, the school:

> shall place a handicapped person in the regular educational environment "unless it is demonstrated" that the education of the person in the regular environment with the use of supplementary aids and services cannot be achieved satisfactorily. (34 C.F.R., Section 104.34 [a], 1998)

Some school districts have formal written procedures for how they identify students, plan for educational accommodations, and implement plans to meet students' needs in compliance with the requirements of Section 504 of the Rehabilitation Act. School districts *may* have a team of people with a coordinator whose responsibility is to evaluate any student who meets the criteria of a "person with a disability" and to determine the student's needs in school— physical and/or educational. When this is the case, the team works with the parents and hopefully agrees or compromises with them on the types of modifications and accommodations their child needs to succeed in school. No law states that this must be the case, and many districts may not even have a specific person who is in charge of the 504 plan. In addition, nothing in the federal law states that it must be a "written" plan. The law is not an education law, but a civil rights law. It was meant to protect students with disabilities from being discriminated against based on their disability and also to ensure they receive a FAPE.

A 504 plan can be as informal as establishing a modified physical education program, or as formal as having transportation services provided and helping to create a detailed outline of services and accommodations for your YPWC (see Appendix H for sample plans). The extent of the accommodations your YPWC needs will depend upon the severity of your child's symptoms, his or her ability to attend school, and your personal feelings. It also depends, in large part, on the willingness of the school staff to work with you to provide the necessary accommodations for your child's academic success.

Whether the school district has formal procedures on how to comply with Section 504 or informal procedures in which the entire evaluation and determination of needs seems haphazard, problems can still arise. Although the right to a 504 plan is guaranteed under Section 504 of the Rehabilitation Act, the way a district sets it up, implements the modifications, and follows through varies from district to district. One common problem is that although there is a plan (hopefully written) in place, it may not be clear as to who is responsible for ensuring the plan is implemented. For example, let us assume that you have a son, Joe, who is allowed to use a calculator in math class and on tests. You find out during the year that he has not been allowed to use it. When you try to determine why, you learn that no one told the teacher he was allowed to use it, as stated in his 504 plan. Naturally, you would think that this should never happen, but in reality, it does.

The advantage of having a 504 plan in place is that it establishes that the school has recognized your YPWC's condition and the need for accommodations in your child's educational program. Let us return to the previously mentioned example of the new principal. In that scenario, if you had had a written 504 plan in place, it would have been easier to ensure your child continued to get the services that had been promised. You have nothing to pass on to the new staff if you have only verbal agreements with the original staff.

It is always to your advantage to document the accommodations and services that you receive from the school. We call it creating a "paper trail." By documenting services in such a manner, you have evidence that the school has acknowledged your child's disability in relation to CFIDS, making it much easier to continue to secure services as needed in the future. Section 504 also addresses procedural safeguards to ensure that your child is identified, evaluated, and receiving services under this act. It also gives parents the opportunity to review relevant records and to establish a review procedure of the child's placement (34 C.F.R., Section 104.36, 1998).

If a parent has a complaint about how the school implements the Section 504 regulations, he or she will be referred to the United States Department of Education, Office for Civil Rights (OCR) (see Appendix E). The OCR staff will investigate the complaint to ensure that the process has been correctly followed, as outlined in the regulations. Their rulings will usually address the school's procedures, not the individual placement of a student.

The Individuals with Disabilities Education Act (IDEA)

The Individuals with Disabilities Education Act—IDEA (20 U.S.C., Section 1400 et seq., 1997), formerly known as the Education of the Handicapped Act—guarantees a free appropriate public education for eligible children and youth with disabilities and outlines these children's rights. Once an education law such as the IDEA becomes federal law, each state then reviews it and develops specific policies for the special education and related services of children with disabilities in that state. The local public school district then uses these state guidelines and refines their policies based on the federal laws and regulations, as well as on the laws and policies defined by the state. Write to your state's Education Department—Special Education Division for a copy of your state's policies (see Appendix E for listing of state education departments). All the rights outlined in the federal rendition of the IDEA are guaranteed; however, your state and/or district may have refined the law to afford you with additional rights.

Many parents who are considering having their child evaluated for special education services do not know where to begin. To qualify for these services, a child must have a disability that is "adversely affecting educational performance." If you believe that your child is struggling at school, you are advised to learn more about the IDEA. An excellent resource, which we encourage you to consult, is NICHCY—National Information Center for Children and Youth with Disabilities—an information clearinghouse that provides information on disabilities and disability-related issues. NICHCY is a project of the Academy for Educational Development, founded in 1961, and is operated through an agreement with the Office of Special Education Programs, U.S. Department of Education. NICHCY has an extensive listing of resources for parents and educators trying to determine how this legislation fits their needs. The center's information is extensive, well referenced, usually in question-and-answer format, and very easy for most parents to understand. Assistance is offered over the phone, via e-mail, or at their Web site (see Appendix E).

As a parent of a YPWC who might benefit from special education services, you may wonder what the IDEA's purpose is. "Questions Often Asked About Special Education Services," a publication of NICHCY, states that the major purposes of the IDEA are to:

1. guarantee the availability of special education programs to eligible children and youth with disabilities;
2. assure that decisions made about providing special education to children and youth with disabilities are fair and appropriate; and
3. financially assist the efforts of state and local governments to educate children with special needs through the use of Federal funds. (NICHCY, 1994)

The IDEA differs from Section 504 in many ways. IDEA is an education law, not a civil rights law. The U.S. Department of Education Office of Special Education and Rehabilitative Services (OSERS), *which is an education agency,* protects a child classified under IDEA (see Appendix E), whereas Section 504 complaints are referred to The U.S. Department of Education, Office for Civil Rights (OCR), a civil rights agency (see Appendix E). Also, schools receive financial assistance under the IDEA to educate classified children with disabilities, which is not available under Section 504.

Students with various types of disabilities are eligible for special education services. A YPWC who is in need of such services would be classified under one of the disabilities listed in the IDEA. The most common classification for the YPWC is "Other Health Impaired." The definition of this disability states:

> "Other health impairment" means having limited strength, vitality or alertness, due to chronic or acute health problems such as a heart condition, tuberculosis, rheumatic fever, nephritis, asthma, sickle cell anemia, hemophilia, epilepsy, lead poisoning, leukemia, or diabetes, that adversely affects a child's educational performance. (34 C.F.R., Section 300.7, 1997)

All possible health conditions are not included in this definition, so as not to exclude illnesses such as CFIDS.

Some parents have negative feelings about their child being classified as a "special education student." One couple in a support group stated that this is how they initially felt about their son:

> We looked at special education as being for severely impaired students with learning disabilities, emotional and/or physical problems. We saw it as the tiny room at the end of the hall where all the children with the problems went who couldn't be taught in the conventional way. We envisioned only the severely impaired and had to get past that stigma to realize that that is a very limited, stereotyped view of what special education really is. By not exploring this option we were actually limiting our son's chances to achieve to his full educational potential.

If your child is able to attend school, he or she could receive the services under the IDEA with the regular education classroom and teacher. A special education teacher, such as a resource room teacher or teacher consultant, would work with the classroom teacher to make any necessary curriculum accommodations and/or modifications for your child. If your child attends school for part of the day, one service could be to provide class time in the resource room for one to two periods. Although the resource room teacher is already working with the classroom teacher, this period would allow your child to have some one-on-one time to improve performance and work on any identified weak skills, such as study, math, or reading skills.

The Individualized Education Program (IEP)

You may be confused at this point. How can you tell if you should request an educational evaluation of your child? Let us look at the following scenario with a seventh grade YPWC named Alex. Alex had suffered from CFIDS for two years but had managed to maintain his grade level in school. Though he was unable to attend school for more than a couple of classes a day, his mother would pick up his assignments to keep him on track with his classmates. However, completing the work took 100 percent of his effort. His parents noticed that it was a greater struggle with every assignment. They had to read the text to him, as he could no longer comprehend it on his own. His skills in math were slowly deteriorating, and working on lengthy assignments would quickly give him a headache. The homework continued to pile up.

Alex was also not benefiting from the teacher's lessons. He was learning the entire course content through homework assignments. Although the intent of homework is to complement and reinforce the concepts taught in the lesson, Alex was using it exclusively to learn the course material. Alex's mom stated:

> If there was just a way to modify these assignments so that he was only doing the really important ones. If we had some course guidelines so that we would know what he is supposed to be mastering, it would help. If he could stop doing worksheets on skills he has mastered, then he could concentrate on the skills that need his attention.

They also learned that some of the projects he was required to do alone had actually been group projects for the students in the class. His parents were worried that if he did not get some help with his lessons and homework, he would soon fall hopelessly behind.

Then they began to ask about possible educational services for their son. They were told that Alex could be evaluated for special education and, if found eligible, would have an Individualized Education Program (IEP) designed just for him. His curriculum would be modified to include attainable goals within the confines of his disability. By breaking down the required curriculum in this manner, he was able to finish the year with flying colors. He was placed in the least restrictive environment (LRE), which was to continue in the same classes with his classmates, but with some homework and testing modifications that made his schoolwork manageable. He also was assigned a home tutor to teach him the course work for the subjects he missed at school.

In placing a child like Alex in the LRE, the Committee on Special Education (CSE) must consider three things. First is the appropriateness of the programs and services for meeting the needs of the student. Second are the opportunities for the child to be educated and involved with nondisabled peers. Finally, the distance between the school and the student's home must be considered.

At this point, if you have decided that your child's CFIDS is adversely affecting his or her educational performance, it is time to request that an educational evaluation be done by the school. It is advised that you make such a request in writing. The letter should be addressed to the principal and/or the CSE chairperson. The letter should be short and should simply state that you would like to refer your child to the CSE. You should ask that they conduct an individual evaluation to determine if an educational disability is present that will make your child eligible for special education services. You should also state your concerns about your child's educational difficulties, for example, in reading comprehension and/or math computation. Request that the school contact you to discuss the referral.

Once the referral has been received, a time line goes into effect. The school must act on the evaluation and notify parents about what is happening, throughout the process. For more detailed information on this component of the Special Education evaluation, your due process rights, and other special education issues, contact your school or state education department for a booklet that outlines the complete process to be followed. You can also contact NICHCY for detailed information on these topics (see Appendix E).

If, following the individual evaluation, your child is found eligible for special education services, then the next phase is to consider what services and accommodations you believe your child needs to succeed in school. You will have an opportunity to share your thoughts with the Committee on Special Education at the IEP meeting to develop your YPWC's Individualized Education Program (IEP).

The most frequent accommodations provided for YPWCs will often involve homework and testing modifications. If your YPWC is not attending school on a full-time basis, he or she will probably have difficulty completing the same amount of homework that is expected of other students. The IEP team may choose to modify the length of the assignments. This will enable your child to demonstrate the acquired skill by doing twenty math problems rather than being "wiped out" by doing the fifty that the class was required to do. Other modifications in homework may include a computer or word processor for a YPWC who has difficulty writing, a calculator for use in math computation, or books on tape when reading comprehension is a problem (see Appendix E for how to secure these special tapes and the tape player needed to play them). Your child may also be allowed modifications on test taking, such as extended time, taking the test in an alternate location, increasing the size of the test questions, limiting the number of questions per page, or having the test read aloud by someone. These are only a few of the accommodations that YPWCs have found helpful.

When you meet with the Committee on Special Education to plan the Individual Education Program (IEP), you will be able to discuss your child's needs and what services and accommodations you feel would help your child to achieve his or her educational potential. As parents, you will most likely be asked to fill out a form or offer ideas on your child's individual characteristics, such as your child's learning styles, social and emotional strengths and needs, and management needs. A special education teacher stressed the importance of this information:

It would be really helpful to YPWCs' teachers if the parents would get very specific under the individual characteristics. For example, what are the child's seating preferences? Would they do better seated up front near the board and the teacher? Does the lighting have an effect on the child's condition? How have the parents found they learn best: flashcards, repetition, hands-on experiences? What cognitive problems have the parents noticed in their learning? Do they have more difficulty doing certain tasks or skills?

This teacher noted that the more specific the parents are at the IEP meeting, the better the teacher understands the child's strengths and weaknesses. Specific information enables the development of an IEP that is truly individualized to your child's needs.

It may be helpful for you to talk to someone prior to this meeting to discuss some possible services and accommodations that would benefit your YPWC. The resource room teacher or guidance counselor may be able to assist you, as well as other parents of YPWCs who are in the same situation.

The IEP obligation in the IDEA has two principal parts as described in the act and regulations:

1. The IEP meeting(s), where decisions are mutually made and agreed to by the parents and school personnel about an educational program for the child with a disability, and
2. The IEP document itself, which is a written record of the decisions reached at the meeting.

When addressing parent participation at IEP meetings, we can look to the IDEA section 300.345, which states that each public agency shall take steps to ensure that one or both of the parents of the child with a disability are present at each meeting or are afforded the opportunity to participate, including:

1. notifying parents of the meeting early enough to ensure that they will have an opportunity to attend; and
2. scheduling the meeting at a mutually agreed upon time and place. (34 C.F.R., Section 300.345, 1996)

At this IEP meeting, the IEP document is developed. The IEP should not be completed and ready for your signature at the beginning of this meeting; it is to be discussed and outlined at this meeting, taking into account the recommendations of the committee and you, the parents. You may wonder what is included in the IEP document. The parts of the IEP are outlined in detail in "Content of Individualized Education Program" (34 C.F.R., Section 300.346, 1996):

Sec. 300.346 Content of individualized education program.

(a) General. The IEP for each child must include—

(1) A statement of the child's present levels of educational performance;

(2) A statement of annual goals, including short-term instructional objectives;

(3) A statement of the specific special education and related services to be provided to the child and the extent that the child will be able to participate in regular educational programs;

(4) The projected dates for initiation of services and the anticipated duration of the services; and

(5) Appropriate objective criteria and evaluation procedures and schedules for determining, on at least an annual basis, whether the short term instructional objectives are being achieved.

(b) Transition services.

(1) The IEP for each student, beginning no later than age 16 (and at a younger age, if determined appropriate), must include a statement of the needed transition services as defined in Sec. 300.18, including, if appropriate, a statement of each public agency's and each participating agency's responsibilities or linkages, or both, before the student leaves the school setting.

(2) If the IEP team determines that services are not needed in one or more of the areas specified in Sec. 300.18 (b)(2)(i) through (b)(2)(iii), the IEP must include a statement to that effect and the basis upon which the determination was made.

(Authority: 20 U.S.C. 1401 (a)(19), (a)(20); 1412 (2)(B), (4), (6); 1414(a) (5))

Some parents of YPWCs find that the inclusion of transition services in the IEP is another reason it is preferable to a 504 plan. These services, not a part of the 504 plan, will aid your child in the transition from high school to the world beyond, be it a postsecondary education, a job, or whatever your child decides to do. The school is required to assist the student with a disability in this planning, taking into consideration any limitations present and accommodations required.

Another advantage to the IEP is the specific due process rights guaranteed the parents. You have the right to disagree and challenge the findings of the CSE in relation to your child's identification, individual evaluation, and the final placement. The school is required to inform you of these rights. NICHCY (see Appendix E) is an excellent place to go if you have any questions on what your rights are or need assistance in ensuring that your rights are met.

The annual goals listed in your child's IEP are statements that describe what your child can realistically be expected to achieve in twelve months in his or her special education program. The annual goals are written after examining your child's present levels of educational performance.

Whereas the annual goals are long-term expectations, the short-term instructional objectives are the steps your child will take to get from the present level of performance to the annual goals in the IEP. The IEP will outline each area of the curriculum in which the disability is affecting the child's involvement and progress. It will list the major goals for your child (annual goals) and then a number of short-term instructional objectives to help your child achieve each of those goals (see Appendix H—sample IEP).

The goals and objectives of the IEP make this plan preferable to a 504 plan. The 504 plans, although offering services and accommodations, do not have goals and objectives. YPWCs who are unable to function at the level of their peers may truly benefit from this individualized curriculum. Children's course requirements will be based on their own personal annual goals and objectives as spelled out in their IEP.

If your child is unable to attend school at all, you can request a home tutor. Regulations regarding home tutors vary from state to state, and district to district. Many do not even address the issue.

However, you have every right to request that the school provide your child with a tutor. If YPWCs are unable to attend school because of this illness, then the least restrictive environment to educate them in would be the home.

The IEP is preferable to the 504 plan if your child is unable to attend school. Whether you have a home tutor or are doing the teaching yourself, it will be far easier to set up lessons and teach the course work with the goals and objectives set forth in the IEP. It provides you with the framework of the curriculum and enables you to see what the expectations are for the year so that you can plan accordingly. This, in itself, can mean all the difference to the home-bound student, making the academic load individualized and manageable.

As parents learn more about the IDEA and think about the services that their YPWC needs to succeed, they begin to feel more confident as their child's advocate. Some will conclude that their child's educational needs can be met under Section 504 by the addition of a few extra services and accommodations (see Appendix H for samples). Other parents will see the need for an IEP for their YPWC to continue to be successful in school. Each situation is different, but what remains the same is that parents must educate themselves and become the advocate their child needs.

Two parents in a support group had this to say about the choices they made for their two YPWCs:

> We found learning more about our children's educational options critical to being able to help them to succeed. One of our YPWCs currently receives services under a 504 plan. While CFIDS does have an impact on our daughter's learning, the accommodations we secured through the school give her the edge she needs to succeed and continue to excel in her schooling. Our other YPWC started out with a 504 plan. As the illness progressed and he was unable to fulfill the requirements in his courses, we were able to secure him services under the IDEA. Having an IEP has made all the difference in the world to him. He is now able to reach his goals with help from the services and accommodations he was guaranteed under the IDEA. For us as parents, this has meant that we are

spending more time supporting our children's achievements than fighting for someone to understand and acknowledge their unique problems. There are still some bumps in the road and hurdles to overcome, but it is now much easier for us all.

We realize that this may be a lot of information for you to digest. If, up to this point, you have been unfamiliar with Section 504 of the Rehabilitation Act or the IDEA, you may feel lost and over-whelmed. Many people have felt this way in the search for the right educational program for their YPWC. It is so important for you to become familiar with the laws and how they pertain to your child. As previously stated, the school should be familiar with these laws, but may not see how they relate to CFIDS. Hopefully, we have addressed a few key points in this chapter that will help you in this task. You may need to keep restating your goals before the school will listen to you. Remember that your child has the right to a free appropriate public education (FAPE) under both section 504 and the IDEA. If your child is not functioning at the level of his or her peers, and CFIDS is affecting his or her academic performance, then you should request an individual education evaluation.

We encourage you to discuss your YPWC's educational options with the personnel at your child's school. We also advise you to learn all that you can about your child's rights and the school's responsibility to ensure them a FAPE. There are parent advocacy groups in most states to assist you in doing just that. Contact your school, your state education department, or NICHCY and request a directory of the resources in your state.

Chapter 9

Evaluating Intellectual Abilities

In this chapter, we will share with you some information on educational testing. If you have requested, or the school has recommended, an educational evaluation, an educational diagnostician will now test and document your child's possible cognitive deficits. This assessment may consist of various tests such as standardized intelligence and/or achievement tests and may be a necessary step toward deciding if your child's educational performance is being adversely affected by CFIDS.

STANDARDIZED TESTS

Standardized testing compares a particular student with a group of similar students. The group is generally a nationwide sample of students at the same grade level as the student being tested. Some tests focus on the elementary levels—first and second grade and third to fifth grade. These tests come in two basic types: one is for use with an individual student, while the second is used with a group of students. Your child may have been given a group test in the past and now be required to take an individual evaluation as a part of assessing his or her need for further academic services. Your child may be required to take two different tests as part of the school's assessment. Both of these tests measure what has been learned and learning potential, but they also each have their own uses. The education evaluator will determine if one or both tests are necessary to fully assess your child's need for further academic services.

Intelligence Tests

Intelligence is the ability to learn and deal with new situations and tasks. The purpose of intelligence testing is to measure a student's ability to do well in the traditional school setting, such as listening to lectures, taking notes, and completing worksheets. A good test will help predict how well a child will do in school by measuring indirect learning. Students must take the information they have learned and apply it to new situations, which requires more skill in abstract reasoning. They may have learned about analogies and must now apply that knowledge on the test, but using shapes, not words. This test enables the evaluator to determine the student's IQ, or intelligence quotient. Intelligence tests do not measure all areas that affect intelligence, such as social skills and artistic or musical ability. For this reason, many companies have changed the name of their tests from "intelligence" to "aptitude or ability" tests.

Achievement Tests

Achievement tests are used to measure the direct learning of specific subject matter. Concrete reasoning skills, rather than abstract, are the focus of these tests. For example, the student may have mastered map reading, certain math computations, and decoding skills in reading, and these particular skills will be tested directly. Standardized achievement tests are more commonly used at the elementary school level, as opposed to the high school level, because the curricula at this level are more consistent throughout the country.

PREPARING FOR TESTING

You should be sensitive to any resistance on the part of your child toward being tested. Your child may be apprehensive about formal testing due to anxiety about increased academic difficulties. Explain to your child that the test results will be used to help identify strengths as well as weaknesses and, in turn, will assist the school personnel in developing teaching strategies to help with his or her schoolwork.

You may choose to meet initially with the evaluator on an individual basis to discuss the testing. At this time, you can share information about cognitive deficits in your child that you have observed. This will help the tester better understand your child's behavior during testing. Although a tester may view the child as being easily distracted and careless, a parent's observations of attending difficulties common to CFIDS will help explain the results and clarify the YPWC's situation.

Testing Conditions

Another factor to consider is that the physical setting for a test administration can affect your child's performance. The evaluation should be given in a room that is free of outside stimuli so that your YPWC is less likely to be distracted. Momentary disruptions may greatly interfere with the YPWC's concentration abilities during testing. Therefore, the evaluator needs to ensure that your child will not be interrupted during testing.

Although adequate lighting is important for all academic testing, the evaluator should be aware that many YPWCs are sensitive to fluorescent lights. Administering the test in a room with proper lighting may actually enhance your child's performance.

INTERPRETING PERFORMANCE

A single test score does not accurately measure all of your child's abilities, including cognitive strengths and weaknesses. There are many other factors that shape intelligence and achievement in children. These include several traits and attitudes such as enthusiasm, anxiety, and persistence. Awareness of these factors may help in planning academic remediation strategies for limitations produced by CFIDS or in developing the best teaching methods to enhance identified strengths. For example, a child's persistence may help him or her deal with the frustration caused by concentration difficulties.

Feedback About Results

Your YPWC's strengths and weaknesses should not be discussed in isolation. It is important for you and the evaluators to stress how your child's personal characteristics, such as motivation and persistence, may help him or her deal with the cognitive limitations.

Together, you can decide whether to include your child in this initial meeting or to have the evaluator explain the results afterward. Help your child to understand his or her scores. Even if children have done as well as expected, the test still should be discussed to emphasize their strengths. Specific strategies for dealing with the cognitive limitations should also be discussed with them. For example, you can tell your child that the evaluator will help teachers understand that his or her performance is unnecessarily affected by time limits. By making the modification of extending time limits for testing and homework assignments your child may be more confident about his or her academic abilities.

The more that you, as parents, understand the entire evaluation process, the more help you will be in advocating for your YPWC. Becoming involved in the planning of your child's educational program is essential to its success. By understanding what the different types of tests are meant to evaluate, you can help choose the areas that need to be addressed in your child's evaluation. You may be able to offer ideas on educational modifications that will enable your child to succeed in school.

Advocacy requires becoming informed and involved about every avenue of your child's education. Parents need to understand their rights and the processes involved in determining eligibility for educational services and accommodations. You must remember that you know your child better than anyone else does, and only you can ensure that your YPWC receives the services needed to succeed.

Epilogue

Look How Far We've Come

In Lyndonville, New York, in 1985, there were many cases of a mononucleosis-like illness that affected over 100 people, several of them children.

This was a very frightening time because of the fear of the unknown. As a parent of four daughters who suddenly became ill within a week's time, I had good reason to be frightened. It became apparent all too quickly that this illness—without a name, without a laboratory marker, without any successful treatment—without knowing if it was fatal—would rule the lives of many people for many years.

Physicians in this country could not provide a valid diagnosis for patients who had this illness because its symptoms did not fit any known medical syndrome. Schools did not have to provide help to families since they could not present medical proof of a real illness. Insurance companies would not recognize this illness because there was no insurance code assigned to it (nothing pertaining to an illness is paid for without a code). And disability insurance was unheard of for people suffering from this illness. Many patients underwent high-risk experimental treatments, muscle biopsies, blood test after blood test, exploratory surgery, CT scans, and MRIs. Although a case control study was done, and subsequently published, it did not determine the cause of the outbreak.

However, most people do not realize how far we have come. This once nameless disease that fit no logical medical syndrome has since been named—chronic fatigue syndrome—and it is not fatal.

Today, fourteen years after the initial outbreak in Lyndonville, much has been learned about this illness. Knowledgeable physicians care about their patients, even if they cannot cure them. Support groups exist in every state and nearly every city. Exclusionary blood tests are available to rule out other illnesses, even if there still is no laboratory marker to pinpoint CFIDS. Many books have been written by physicians and patients. Money is being awarded to research projects all over the United States. Conferences are held almost every year to share information from all over the world. Many patients have been awarded disability compensation. Many schools work with students who are ill and cannot attend full-time. Each YPWC is an important, unique, and special individual who has the right to develop to his or her fullest potential. Although it may be overwhelming at times, it is worth the effort to keep your child's name and face in front of the teachers and to do everything in your power to guarantee your child receives the best that the school has to offer. This is the reason this guide was created—to share what we have learned through our research and personal trials and tribulations. Though difficult at times, parents the world over have managed to become the advocates that their children needed at a time in their lives when they could not have managed it alone.

Certainly, we have far to go. But look how far we have come!

Jean Pollard

APPENDIXES

Appendix A

Chronic Fatigue Immune Dysfunction Syndrome (CFIDS) Health Questionnaire for School Personnel

(The following is a questionnaire that may be used by teachers, parents, and/or health care professionals to assist in the diagnosis of CFIDS in the school-age child.)

		YES	NO
1.	Did the illness begin with a sudden onset such as flu or mono-like infection?	____	____
2.	Since the onset, has there been a single week during which you felt entirely well?	____	____
3.	Does the fatigue go away with a good night's sleep?	____	____
4.	Do you have trouble getting a refreshing night's sleep?	____	____
5.	Do you feel fatigued every day?	____	____
6.	Does exertion or activity make the fatigue worse?	____	____
7.	Do you have a sore throat at least once a week?	____	____
8.	Are the glands in your neck frequently sore?	____	____
9.	Does light hurt your eyes?	____	____
10.	Does noise make you uncomfortable?	____	____
11.	Are you bothered by odors?	____	____

12. Do you have pain in your stomach more than once a week? _____ _____

13. Do you experience muscle pain? _____ _____

14. Do your muscles ever feel weak? _____ _____

15. Do you experience joint (knee, ankle, finger, etc.) pain? _____ _____

16. Do you get headaches more than once or twice a week? _____ _____

17. Do you have difficulty concentrating? _____ _____

18. Is it difficult for you to remember simple things? _____ _____

19. Do you often feel light-headed and dizzy? _____ _____

20. Do you frequently feel like you have a fever? _____ _____

21. Do you experience night sweats? _____ _____

Totals: _____ _____

Measuring the Child's Overall Activity Limitations

On an average day, how many hours are spent engaged in each of the following activities (total number of hours should equal twenty-four): (Note: hours sleeping do not have to be all at once, but over a twenty-four-hour period.)

a. Sleeping: _____

b. Resting, but not sleeping: _____

c. Light activities while sitting or lying down (watching TV, recreational reading, etc.): _____

d. Moderate activities around the house (home tutoring, studying, meals, doing chores, etc.): _____

e. Moderate activities outside of the house (school, walking, shopping, etc.): _____

f. Vigorous activity (exercise, biking, sports, heavy cleaning, etc.): _____

Total: 24

Answers Commonly Heard from Moderately Ill YPWCs

1. Yes—70 percent have sudden onset, while 30 percent have gradual onset.
2. No.
3. Almost never—sleep difficulties always take place as either insomnia, unrefreshing sleep, or sleeping late in the morning.

4-21. Generally yes.

Measurement of overall activity limitation compares the number of hours of inactivity (a, b, c) to the number of hours of activity (d, e, f). For example:

- A typical day for a healthy child is roughly twelve hours of activity and twelve hours of inactivity.
- For the YPWC, you usually see fewer than eight hours of activity, and none of it is vigorous (f).
- A severe case of CFIDS usually involves fewer than four hours of activity.

Appendix B

Chronic Fatigue Immune Dysfunction (CFIDS) Organizations and National Support Groups

American Association for Chronic Fatigue Syndrome (AACFS)
7 Van Buren Street
Albany, NY 12206
(518) 482-2202; (518) 435-1765 (fax)
e-mail: LBAACFS@AOL.COM
Web site: http://weber.u.washington.edu/~dedra/aacfs1.html

The AACFS is a nonprofit organization for research scientists, physicians, licensed medical health care professionals, and other individuals and institutions interested in promoting the stimulation, coordination, and exchange of ideas for CFS research and patient care, as well as providing periodic reviews of current clinical, research, and treatment ideas on CFS for the benefit of CFS patients and others.

Contact any of the following national support groups for a listing of state and/or local CFIDS support groups. Also, request a listing of their publications, which are too numerous to include here.

National CFIDS Foundation
103 Aletha Road
Needham, MA 02192
(617) 449-3535
e-mail: gailronda@aol.com
Web site: http://www.cfidsfoundation.org

The National CFIDS Foundation is a nonprofit charitable organization whose goals are to further research and help patients with CFIDS/FMS and related disorders by dispensing accurate information via their quarterly newsletter. Volunteers run the organization, and all money not used for the minimal operating expenses goes directly to fund research. Among the CFIDS brochures and information they distribute, they have a children's packet of information on CFIDS, and also an educational packet to assist in communication with the school.

National CFS and Fibromyalgia Association
P.O. Box 18426
Kansas City, MO 64133
(816) 313-2000 (voice)
e-mail: KEAL55A@prodigy.com
Web site:
http://www.social.com/health/nhic/data/hr2400/hr2415.html

The National Chronic Fatigue Syndrome and Fibromyalgia Association is a nonprofit voluntary organization formed to educate and inform the public, patients and their families, and health professionals about the nature and impact of chronic fatigue syndrome (CFS) and related disorders, including chronic fatigue and immune dysfunction syndrome, chronic Epstein-Barr virus, and myalgic encephalomyelitis. Services include response to inquiries about the condition, educational and resource materials, and referrals to physicians and support groups. The organization also encourages legislative and private funding for research. The primary focus of the association is on scientifically accurate information.

The CFIDS Association of America
P.O. Box 220398
Charlotte, NC 28222-0398
(800) 442-3437 (24-hour voice information line)
e-mail: cfids@cfids.org
Web site: http://www.cfids.org

The CFIDS Association of America, Inc., is a public, nonprofit, charitable organization. They publish a journal titled *The CFIDS Chronicle.* The association directly funds CFIDS research and advocacy efforts and provides information about CFIDS to all who inquire. They have an extensive list of educational materials available on many aspects of CFIDS.

CFIDS Youth Alliance
P.O. Box 220398
Charlotte, NC 28222-0398
(800) 442-3437 (24-hour voice information line)

e-mail: cya@cfids.org
Web site: http://www.cfids.org/cya

CYA is dedicated to increasing advocacy, information, research, and encouragement for persons with CFIDS, ages twenty-four and younger. The CYA Pen Pal Connection matches YPWCs, parents, and siblings with their peers to encourage mutual support and learning.

CFS & FMS Teen Voices

c/o Jennifer Day
205 Walnut Street
Red Oak, IA 51566
Jen's e-mail: jennyd@redoak.heartland.net
Jen's CFIDS Homepage:
Web site: http://www.geocities.com/Heartland/Meadows/7739

CFS & FMS Teen Voices is a national newsletter for YPWCs and their families or loved ones. It discusses the topics that most YPWCs face every day and helps them by lending support and advice. It is published by two teenage YPWCs, Connie Howard and Jennifer Day. A subscription includes six issues (bimonthly) for $8 U.S. or $12 overseas. If you would like a sample issue of the newsletter for YPWCs, please send $.55. For a subscription, please send checks made out to Jennifer Day for the amount due.

Appendix C

On-Line Resources

The Internet has many resources available that pertain to CFIDS. Some sites offer general information about CFIDS, and others, known as newsgroups, post messages and feelings pertaining to this illness. See Appendix B for Web sites of national support groups.

1. CFS Information Resource—includes countless links to other Web sites dealing with CFS information, on-line resources, and more. An excellent choice: http://www.cais.com/cfs-news
2. A youth Web site—with parents' section—YPWCnet: http://www.ypwcnet.org/
3. Directory of support groups: http://www.theriver.com/Public/cfids/
4. ME—Web resource page in the Netherlands: http://www.dds.nl/~me-net/meweb
5. United Kingdom—ME site: http://www.community-care.org.uk/ME/
6. List of CFIDS-related e-mail groups, includes particular interest of participants and how to sign up: http://members.aol.com/cfslists/lists.htm
7. List of CFIDS discussion groups: http://www.cais.com/cfs-news/index.htm#TALKGeneral CFS resources
8. *CFS-NEWS* is an electronic newsletter available at no cost through e-mail. To get on the *CFS-NEWS* mailing list, create an e-mail message, that says SUB CFS-NEWS YourFirstName YourLastName (but use your own name) and send to LISTSERV@MAELSTROM. STJOHNS.EDU. Do not put anything else in the body of your message. It must be exactly as stated here.
9. Web site for Parents of Sick and Worn-Out Kids: http://www.bluecrab.org/health/sickids/sickids.htm
10. CFS on-line newsletter by Dr. Bell and Associates that discusses current research, adult and pediatric issues related to CFS, Q&A section, and more. For information, direct e-mail to: CFS-DSBELL @juno.com and put NEWSLETTER in the subject box.

Appendix D

Letters to the School from the Physician

Letter # 1

Date
Name, CSE Chairperson
Central Schools
City, State, Zip
Dear _____, CSE Chairperson:

This letter is in regard to *child's name* who has been diagnosed with Chronic Fatigue Immune Dysfunction Syndrome and has been followed in this office for the past *number* years. *His or her* primary symptoms include severe abdominal pain, muscle and joint pain, sore throats, fatigue, difficulty sleeping, and cognitive problems *(list child's major symptoms)*.

Child's name clearly has a medical condition that is interfering with *his or her* educational performance. This "other health impairment" is characterized by "limited strength, decreased alertness and vitality," and cognitive difficulties that impair *his or her* ability to attend school and to learn through normal teaching methods. *Child's name's* cognitive impairments include inability to concentrate, short-term memory impediments, word finding difficulties, deficits in mathematical computation, and problems with visual spatial perception *(list child's major cognitive symptoms)*.

For *child's name* to be able to reach *his or her* educational potential, I feel that *he or she* needs special accommodations from the school. We will attempt to increase the amount of time that *he or she* can spend at the school, depending upon the severity of *his or her* symptoms. However, *he or she* will need home tutoring, as *he or she* is not able to attend school on a full-time basis. Other suggested accommodations that are needed: testing modifications, homework and classwork modifications, books on tape, use of a calculator, word processor, and a tape recorder *(list those that apply)*.

I would like to make a referral for physical therapy due to *child's name's* limited strength, mobility, and endurance within the educational setting. These physical problems and the accompanying pain limit *his or her* ability to function in a regular classroom setting. It is hoped that physical therapy will improve *his or her* independence and allow greater attendance in school.

Very truly yours,

David S. Bell, MD

Letter #2

Date
Name, School Principal
Address
Dear _____:

Due to *child's name's* continuing symptoms of chronic fatigue immune dysfunction syndrome, it is my recommendation that he or she attend school for one to two hours per day and receive one hour of tutoring a day to make up the remainder of the curriculum. I would also strongly recommend no physical education at this time.

If you have any specific questions, please feel free to contact me.

Very truly yours,

David S. Bell, MD

Appendix E

Educational Resources

NICHCY—National Information Center for Children and Youth with Disabilities
P.O. Box 1492
Washington, DC 20013-1492
(800) 695-0285
e-mail: nichcy@aed.org
Web site: http://www.nichcy.org

NICHCY is an information clearinghouse that provides information on disabilities and disability-related issues. Children and youth with disabilities are their special focus. NICHCY is a project of the Academy for Educational Development, founded in 1961, and is operated through an agreement with the Office of Special Education Programs, U.S. Department of Education. NICHCY has an extensive listing of resources that are well referenced and very easy for parents to understand.

HEATH—National Clearinghouse for People with Disabilities Pursuing Education or Training After High School
One Dupont Circle—Suite 800
Washington, DC 20036
(202) 939-9320
e-mail: heath@ace.nche.edu
Web site: http://www.acenet.edu

Recording for the Blind & Dyslexic
20 Roszel Road
Princeton, NJ 08540
(800) 221-4792; (609) 987-8116 (fax)
Web site: http://www.rfbd.org

Recording for the Blind & Dyslexic (RFB&D) is a national nonprofit organization. They provide on loan recorded books at all academic levels for anyone with a documented print-related disability. This includes anyone with a visual, perceptual, or other physical disability that limits his or her effective use of standard print. To document your disability, your application form must be signed by a qualified professional in disability services, education, medicine, or psychology. There is a one-time registration fee and a nominal yearly membership fee for this service. You have the choice of an individual membership, or a school "institutional" membership. Contact RFB&D for more information on both. RFB&D will provide your child with all the needed textbooks on tape, for the year, and will record any books they do not have on tape. If you do not choose to purchase the special tape players from RFB&D that are needed to play these four-track tapes see the following reference to NLS.

National Library Service for the Blind and Physically Handicapped (NLS)

Library of Congress
Washington, DC 20542
Web site: http://www.loc.gov/nls

The National Library Service for the Blind and Physically Handicapped (NLS), Library of Congress, administers a free national library program of braille and recorded materials for blind and physically handicapped persons. Reading materials and playback machines are sent to borrowers at no cost and returned to libraries by postage-free mail. Playback equipment is loaned free to readers for as long as recorded materials provided by NLS and its cooperating libraries are being borrowed. Anyone who is unable to read or use standard printed materials because of temporary or permanent visual or physical limitations may receive these services. You may ask your local public librarian for more information about the program and how to apply for service.

The United States Department of Education, Office for Civil Rights (OCR)

1100 Pennsylvania Avenue, NW Room 316
Washington, DC 20044-4620
(202) 208-2545

The United States Department of Education,
  Office of Special Education and Rehabilitative Services (OSERS)
Mary E. Switzer Building, Room 3123
330 C Street, SW
Washington, DC 20202
(202) 205-8241
Web site: http://www.ed.gov/index.html

State Departments of Education: Special Education

Alabama

Bill East, Director
AL Department of Education,
Division of Special Education Services
P.O. Box 302101
Montgomery, AL 36130-2101
(334) 242-8114; (800) 392-8020 (in AL)

Alaska

DiAnn Brown, Program Manager
Office of Special Education
AK Department of Education
801 West Tenth Street, Suite 200
Juneau, AK 99801-1894
(907) 465-2972

Arizona

Kathryn A. Lund, State Director
Exceptional Student Services, Department of Education
1535 West Jefferson
Phoenix, AZ 85007
(602) 542-3084
e-mail: klund@mail1.ade.state.az.us
URL: http://ade.state.az.us

Arkansas

Diane Sydoriak, Associate Director
Special Education Unit, Department of Education
Special Education Building C, Room 105
#4 Capitol Mall
Little Rock, AR 72201-1071
(501) 682-4225

California

Leo Sandoval, Director
Special Education, Department of Education
515 L Street, Suite 270
Sacramento, CA 95814
(916) 445-4729

Colorado

Lorrie Harkness, Director
Special Education Services Unit
CO Department of Education
201 East Colfax Avenue
Denver, CO 80203
(303) 866-6694

Connecticut

Leslie Averna, Acting Bureau Chief
Bureau of Special Education and Pupil Services
CT Department of Education
25 Industrial Park Road
Middletown, CT 06457-1520
(860) 638-4265

Delaware

Martha Brooks, Team Leader
Exceptional Children and Early Childhood Education
Department of Public Instruction
P.O. Box 1402
Dover, DE 19903
(302) 739-5471

District of Columbia

Jeff Myers, Director
Goding Elementary School
920 F Street, NE
Washington, DC 20002
(202) 724-7833

Florida

Instructional Support and Community Services
Department of Education
325 West Gaines Street, Suite 614
Tallahassee, FL 32399-0400
(904) 488-1570

Georgia

Paulette Bragg, Director
Division for Exceptional Students
GA Department of Education
1870 Twin Towers East
Atlanta, GA 30334
(404) 656-3963

Hawaii

Doug Houck, Administrator
Special Education Section
HI Department of Education
3430 Leahi Avenue
Honolulu, HI 96815
(808) 733-4990

Idaho

Nolene Weaver, Supervisor
Special Education Section
ID Department of Education
P.O. Box 83720
Boise, ID 83720-0027
(208) 332-6917
e-mail: nbweaver@sde.state.id.us

Illinois

Jack Shook, Division Administrator
Center for Educational Innovation and Reform
Program Compliance
100 North First Street, E-228
Springfield, IL 62777-0001
(217) 782-5589

Indiana

Robert Marra, Director
Division of Special Education, Department of Education
State House, Room 229
Indianapolis, IN 46204-2798
(317) 232-0570
e-mail: MARRAB@speced.state.in.us
URL: http://www.indstate.edu/seas/dse.html

Iowa

Jeananne Hagen, Bureau Chief
Bureau of Special Education
IA Department of Education
Grimes State Office Building
Des Moines, IA 50319-0146
(515) 281-5735
e-mail: jhagen@max.state.ia.us

Kansas

Michael Remus, Team Leader
Student Support Services
Kansas State Department of Education
120 East Tenth Street
Topeka, KS 66612
(785) 291-3097
e-mail: mremus@smptgw.ksbe.state.ks.us

Kentucky

Mike Armstrong, Director
Division of Exceptional Children's Services
Kentucky Department of Education
Capitol Plaza Tower, Eighth Floor
Frankfort, KY 40601
(502) 564-4970

Louisiana

Dr. Leon Borne Jr., Assistant Superintendent
Office of Special Educational Services
Louisiana State Department of Education
P.O. Box 94064
Baton Rouge, LA 70804-9064
(504) 342-3633

Maine

David Noble Stockford, Director
Division of Special Education, Department of Education
State House, Station #23
Augusta, ME 04333-0023
(207) 287-5950

Maryland

Beatrice Rodgers, Director
Governor's Office for Individuals with Disabilities
One Market Center, Box 10
300 West Lexington Street
Baltimore, MD 21201-3435
(410) 333-3098 (V/TTY)

Massachusetts

Marcia Mittnacht, Executive Director
Educational Improvement Group
Department of Education
350 Main Street
Malden, MA 02148-5023
(617) 388-3300

Michigan

Richard Baldwin, State Director
Office of Special Education Services
Department of Education
P.O. Box 30008
Lansing, MI 48909-7508
(517) 373-9433

Minnesota

Wayne Erickson, Director
Minnesota Department of Children, Families and Learning
Office of Special Education
811 Capitol Square Building, 550 Cedar Street
St. Paul, MN 55101
(612) 296-1793

Mississippi

Carolyn Black, State Director
Office of Special Education, Department of Education
P.O. Box 771
Jackson, MS 39205-0771
(601) 359-3490

Missouri

Melodie Friedebach, Coordinator
Division of Special Education
Department of Elementary and Secondary Education
P.O. Box 480
Jefferson City, MO 65102
(573) 751-2965

Montana

Robert Runkel, Director
Special Education Division
Office of Public Instruction
P.O. Box 202501
Helena, MT 59620-2501
(406) 444-4429

Nebraska

Gary M. Sherman, Director
Special Populations, Department of Education
P.O. Box 94987
Lincoln, NE 68509-4987
(402) 471-2471 (V/TTY); (402) 471-0117
e-mail: gary_s@nde4.nde.state.ne.us
URL: http://www.nde.state.ne.us/SPED/sped.html

New Hampshire

Robert T. Kennedy, Administrator of Special Education
New Hampshire Department of Education
101 Pleasant Street
Concord, NH 03301-3860
(603) 271-3842

New Jersey

Barbara Gantwerk, Director
Office of Special Education Program, Department of Education
100 Riverview Plaza, P.O. Box 500
Trenton, NJ 08625-0500
(609) 292-0147

New Mexico

Diego Gallegos, State Director
Special Education, Department of Education
Education Building
300 Don Gaspar Avenue
Santa Fe, NM 87501-2786
(505) 827-6541

New York

Lawrence Gloeckler, Deputy Commissioner
Office of Vocational and Educational Services
for Individuals with Disabilities
1 Commerce Plaza, Room 1606
Albany, NY 12234
(518) 474-2714

North Carolina

E. Lowell Harris, Director
Exceptional Children Division
Department of Public Instruction
301 North Wilmington Street, Education Building, #570
Raleigh, NC 27601-2825
(919) 715-1565

North Dakota

Brenda K. Oas, Director
Special Education, Department of Public Instruction
600 East Boulevard Avenue
Bismarck, ND 58505-0440
(701) 328-2277

Nevada

Gloria Dopf, Director
Educational Equity, Department of Education
700 East Fifth Street, Suite 113
Carson City, NV 89701-5096
(702) 687-9142

Ohio

John Herner, Director
Division of Special Education
OH Department of Education
933 High Street
Worthington, OH 43085-4017
(614) 466-2650

Oklahoma

Darla Griffin, Executive Director
Special Education Services, Department of Education
2500 North Lincoln Boulevard
Oklahoma City, OK 73105-4599
(405) 521-3351

Oregon

Steven B. Johnson, Associate Superintendent
Office of Special Education
Department of Education
255 Capitol Street NE
Salem, OR 97310-0203
(503) 378-3598, ext. 639
e-mail: steve.johnson@state.or.us
URL: http://www.ode.state.or.us

Pennsylvania

William W. Penn, EdD, Director
Bureau of Special Education, Department of Education
333 Market Street, Seventh Floor
Harrisburg, PA 17126-0333
(717) 783-2311

Rhode Island

Robert M. Pryhoda, Director
Office of Special Needs
Department of Education, Shepard Building
255 Westminster Street, Room 400
Providence, RI 02903-3400
(401) 277-4600, ext. 2301

South Carolina

Ora Spann, Director
State Department of Education
Office of Programs for Exceptional Children
1429 Senate Street, Room 808
Columbia, SC 29201
(803) 734-8806
e-mail: ospann@sde.state.sc.us

South Dakota

Deborah Barnett, Director
Office of Special Education
700 Governors Drive
Pierre, SD 57501-2291
(605) 773-3678

Tennessee

Joseph Fisher, Executive Director
Division of Special Education
Department of Education
Andrew Johnson Tower, Fifth Floor
710 James Robertson Parkway
Nashville, TN 37243-0380
(615) 741-2851

Texas

Gene Lenz, Senior Director
Texas Education Agency
Division of Special Education
1701 North Congress Avenue
Austin, TX 78701-1494
(512) 463-9414

Utah

Mae Taylor, Director
At Risk and Special Education Services
State Office of Education
250 East 500 South
Salt Lake City, UT 84111-3204
(801) 538-7706

Vermont

Dennis Kane, Director
Family and Educational Support Team
120 State Street, State Office Building
Montpelier, VT 05620-2501
(802) 828-3130

Virginia

H. Douglas Cox, Director
Office of Special Education and Student Services
Department of Education
P.O. Box 2120
Richmond, VA 23218-2120
(804) 225-2402
e-mail: dougcox@pen.k12.va.us

Washington

Douglas Gill, Director
Special Education Section
Superintendent of Public Instruction
P.O. Box 47200
Olympia, WA 98504-7200
(360) 753-6733

West Virginia

Michael A. Valentine, Director
Office of Special Education
Department of Education
1900 Kanawha Boulevard East
Building 6, Room B-304
Charleston, WV 25305
(304) 558-2696

Wisconsin

Juanita S. Pawlisch, Assistant State Superintendent
Paul Halverson, Director
Division for Learning Support: Equity and Advocacy
125 South Webster Street, P.O. Box 7841
Madison, WI 53707-7841
(608) 266-1649; (800) 441-4563
URL: http://www.dpi.state.wi.us/dpi/dlsea/een

Wyoming

Patti J. Muhlenkamp, Director
Department of Education, Special Programs Unit
Hathaway Building, Second Floor
2300 Capitol Avenue
Cheyenne, WY 82002
(307) 777-7417
e-mail: pmuhle@educ.state.wy.us
URL: http://www.k12.wy.us

Appendix F

List of Abbreviations/Acronyms

Abbreviations/Acronyms	Educational/Legal
504	Rehabilitation Act of 1973 (Public Law 93-112, Section 504)
504 Plan	Section 504 Accommodation Plan
CFR	Code of Federal Regulations
CSE	Committee on Special Education
FAPE	Free Appropriate Public Education
FERPA	Family Educational Rights and Privacy Act of 1974—"Buckley Amendment"
IDEA	Individuals with Disabilities Education Act
IEP	Individualized Educational Program
IQ	Intelligence Quotient
LRE	Least Restrictive Environment
USC	United States Code
	Dealing with CFIDS
CFIDS	Chronic Fatigue Immune Dysfunction Syndrome
CFS	Chronic Fatigue Syndrome
PWC	Person with CFIDS
YPWC	Young Person with CFIDS

Abbreviations/Acronyms	Medical Terminology
DX	Diagnosis
RX	Take
ins	At Bedtime
ac	Before Meals
po	By Mouth
tab	Tablet
qd	Every Day
tid	Three Times a Day
disp #60	Dispense 60 Pills
c	With
prn	As Needed
q4h	Every Four Hours
caps	Capsules
bid	Twice a Day
qid	Four Times a Day
pc	After Meals

Appendix G

Seventy-Five Tips for Coping with CFIDS in Children— From Pain to Schoolwork

Medicines

1. Talk to your physician about medicines to help ease your YPWC's pain. Aspirin, Tylenol (acetaminophen), or Advil (ibuprofen) are not the same medicine. Your YPWC may also benefit from other medications available by prescription.
2. To remember when it is time to take medicine, set a timer.
3. YPWCs can check off a box on daily charts after taking their medicine. This helps them to gain some independence and to have some control over this illness.
4. Fill pill cases weekly to remember all medicines. You may choose to use different color pillboxes for a.m./p.m. medicines.
5. Tips to use to make swallowing pills easier:

   a. Crush the pills and put them in liquid or pudding. (Check with your pharmacist first to make sure the medication can be taken with food.)
   b. Using a long, narrow-neck, soft drink bottle to put some liquid in, place the pills on your child's tongue and have him or her drink from the bottle. When drinking from the bottle, the mouth conforms around the tiny opening, and as the liquid rushes up the neck of the bottle and into the mouth, it goes quickly down the throat, taking any pills in the mouth with it. (Believe me—it works!!)
   c. Some drugstores have pill glasses with a slot near the rim to put the pill in. The liquid then carries the pill into the mouth with the beverage. (The slot must be dry to work.)
   d. Ask if there is a liquid or chewable form for the medicine.

Pain Relief

6. For eye pain, buy lightly tinted sunglasses that can be worn to school and that look more like regular glasses.
7. Use a heatable eye mask to help with eye pain/headaches.
8. Cold juices and popsicles may ease sore throats.
9. For nausea or upset stomachs, try ginger ale, Coca-Cola Classic, or flavored ice.
10. Pretzels and crackers may also ease upset stomachs.
11. Buy loose-fitting knit or sweat pants several sizes too big for YPWCs suffering from abdominal pain. Soft cotton fabrics may be better on irritated or sensitive skin.
12. Aspercreme/Sportscreme is helpful for sore muscles and joints. These are now available in aloe-based gels.
13. A heating pad may ease the pain from sore muscles.
14. Ice packs can also soothe sore muscles.
15. Try gel insoles in shoes to comfort the feet when walking.
16. Help your child do gentle stretches to keep the muscles and joints flexible. A physical therapy evaluation is a good way to get professional advice on how to prevent deconditioned muscles within the confines of CFIDS.
17. Some YPWCs may benefit from a "myofacial release" massage given by trained physical therapists or massage therapists.
18. A warm bath at bedtime can soothe overall aches and pains and help the body to relax for sleep.
19. Bath salts may help soothe sore muscles. Bath oil or oatmeal-based soaks may help itchy skin.
20. Learn more about pain management by reading books such as *A Child in Pain,* by childhood pain management expert, Leora Kuttner, PhD, by Hartley & Marks Publishers. Call (800) 277-5887 for information on this book.

For Independence and Mobility

21. Help your child to be independent by getting him or her a cane/crutches/wheelchair/knee braces, whatever it takes so he or she can still move around, even when too achy to do so unassisted.
22. If walking distances is difficult for your child, get a handicap permit for your car.
23. Help your child conserve energy by providing wrist splints and/or arm rests for the computer.

24. Help to keep your child independent by installing a shower seat, handheld showerhead, or a bar to grasp in the shower, if needed. For children with neurally mediated or orthostatic hypotension, heat can exacerbate symptoms.
25. Help your YPWC establish some routines for personal hygiene: brushing teeth, combing hair, washing up.
26. Allow your YPWC to develop his or her own personal style: hairstyles, clothing, makeup.
27. Help your YPWC set personal daily goals. This will give him or her a sense of accomplishment. Encourage your YPWC to tackle difficult tasks when individual energy levels are highest.

Memory

28. Use a large calendar to record all family appointments and a personal date keeper for your YPWC.
29. Give your YPWC a good supply of Post-It notes, a memo mate, or a small tape recorder for help remembering those little things.
30. Your YPWC can use index cards to write down directions, with pictures and landmarks, to frequently traveled places, by foot, bike, or car.
31. Rearrange things in the kitchen and bathroom cupboards so your YPWC can find frequently used items easily.

Relaxation: Rest and Sleep

32. Make your own relaxation tape with your YPWC's favorite music. You could even do a relaxation narrative with the child or parent's voice.
33. Give your YPWC lots of physical contact: body rubs, touching, holding.
34. Always keep a set of headphones and a cassette player by the YPWC's nightstand with tapes to listen to at night. Classical music, stories on tapes, and soothing tunes are all good choices.
35. A white noise machine in the bedroom may assist your YPWC with sleeping.
36. A cool mist humidifier may make it easier for your YPWC to sleep when the air is dry in the room or he or she is experiencing congestion due to allergies.
37. If allergies are a problem, buy nonallergic bedding and pillow covers.

38. Some YPWCs are comforted by long, body pillows while sleeping.
39. Some YPWCs benefit from sleeping in waterbeds.
40. Set aside a regular rest period for the child who does not nap. It can be a ten- to twenty-minute down time to sit and read together, listen to music, or talk.

For the Homebound or Limited YPWC

41. Encourage your child to get dressed every day if he or she can. This helps him or her feel better psychologically.
42. A change of scenery is important to the YPWC, and just going from the bedroom to the living room during the day can help. Keeping the bed for sleeping may also make it easier for the YPWC to sleep.
43. Homebound YPWCs who are not up to getting dressed can at least have "day" pajamas. These should be fancy PJs that are comfortable for lounging and give the feeling of being dressed.
44. Plan outings for your child even if it is just to Grandma's, the store, or the library. The walls begin to close in after a while on everyone. For the adolescent who needs to become more independent, this can be especially distressing.
45. Rent funny movies and tape funny shows. It is very important to find opportunities to laugh.
46. Help your YPWC develop a hobby, such as collecting stamps, stickers, dolls, superhero figures, sports cards, anything he or she enjoys.
47. Provide your YPWC with the opportunity to exercise his or her mind with puzzles, reading, or listening to someone read educational material or some kind of literature.
48. Provide drawing materials and new pads of paper for your YPWC to use to express his or her feelings. New art supplies are always fun for those who enjoy drawing or doodling.
49. Provide your YPWC with a lap desk that can hold frequently used materials.

Emotional Health

50. Provide a journal and encourage your YPWC to write down his or her feelings/fears/frustrations/joys and/or triumphs. (This can also be done on a computer.) Reassure your YPWC that this writing is private and only for his or her eyes to see.
51. Have your child make a list of all the things for which he or she is thankful. This is something you can both add to on a daily or weekly basis.

52. Both YPWCs and caregivers should applaud themselves for their efforts, even if the results are not always consistent or predictable.
53. Focus on the quality in your achievements, not the quantity.

Maintaining Contact and Freedom

54. Get call waiting on your telephone so you will not miss important calls.
55. Install an answering machine so you will not miss calls when attending to your child's needs.
56. Consider getting a cellular phone or pager so you can have the freedom to leave the house while your YPWC is at school or elsewhere.
57. YPWCs may also take the cellular phone when going out for walks and then call if they just cannot walk any farther, or if they are somewhere and need help. It is a remarkable way to give some freedom back to the YPWC and the caregiver.
58. Do not be afraid to ask for help when needed (for both the child and the parent).

Helping the YPWC Organize Schoolwork

Maintaining a sense of order in our lives can improve coping skills, especially in regard to school. Mornings are commonly not a good time of day for the YPWC, making it difficult for him or her to get up and go to school. Through better organizing, this task may become easier. See the following tips:

59. Designate a place to do schoolwork. A desk or table in a quiet corner, or a room that is set up just for lessons and homework, will do nicely.
60. Keep pens, pencils, erasers, pencil sharpeners, crayons, colored pencils, markers, notebook paper, ruler, calculator, and other needed supplies there at all times.
61. The desk should be kept organized at all times to assist the YPWC in maintaining a sense of order in academics. Maintaining the same sense of order at home will assist the YPWC in doing so at school and will help him or her to feel more in control of at least this aspect of life.
62. Supplying a shelf for textbooks, dictionaries, and other school resources in this area will also be useful.

63. If the child has a room or an area with wall space, he or she and the tutor (if there is one) can decorate it with maps, study cards, etc., personalizing this area as the "home learning center."

64. It is advisable to have your child do all his or her schoolwork/homework in this area. It will help him or her associate the desk with mental activity.

65. On occasion, if your child is unable to sit up, doing work on a couch or another area free of distractions is better than not doing the work at all.

66. Assist your YPWC to keep schoolwork organized by purchasing different colored pocket folders for each subject area. Some homebound YPWCs have one folder that they use to transport all completed assignments to school.

67. Purchase a bookbag with sturdy, padded shoulder straps for your YPWC. Keep school supplies in the bookbag so it is always stocked and ready to go.

68. By having a set of textbooks at home, the YPWC can greatly lessen the load that must be carried to and from school.

69. Before turning in each night, gather all school supplies together in one place, preferably the bookbag. If your YPWC goes to school in the morning, it will be much easier not having to search for assignments and supplies.

70. Always having the bookbag packed and ready to go and stored in the same place expedites getting ready in the morning, especially if attendance has been sporadic.

71. Encourage your child to get his or her work done in a timely fashion and to do a little something each day. If he or she knows a report is due in two weeks, the process will be much easier if done in tiny increments rather than all at once.

72. Devote part of each day to schoolwork. The brain should have some mental activity every day if possible.

73. Try to establish a routine for your child in terms of school activities. Set times for school, tutoring, and homework help your child's mind to be better prepared to work each day.

74. Make flashcards to practice vocabulary words or any facts and definitions that must be memorized.

75. If your child uses books on tape, he or she can improve retention of the material by listening to the tape while following the words with his or her eyes and a finger. This creates three memory pathways in the brain from which this information can be recalled when needed.

Appendix H

Sample 504 Plans and IEP

CENTRAL SCHOOL DISTRICT
SECTION 504
STUDENT ACCOMMODATION PLAN

Student _____ Grade __7__ DOB _____

School _____ Date of Meeting _____

1. Describe the nature of the concern:
   "Student's Name" has been diagnosed as having Chronic Fatigue Immune Dysfunction Syndrome (CFIDS), which is recognized as a debilitating medical condition.

2. Describe the basis for the determination of handicap (if any):
   "Student's Name"'s diagnosis has been made by Dr. David Bell, a medical expert on CFIDS.

3. Describe how the handicap affects a major life activity:
   "Student's Name" is unable to attend school for a full day and/or on a regular basis. His or her academic program is limited and determined by his or her daily health status.

4. Describe the reasonable accommodations that are necessary:
   a. Home tutoring: 2 hours/day for 5 days/week
   b. Books on tape

Author's note: Although the following academic plans were actually written for YPWCs, any identifying names and dates have been changed to protect their privacy.

143

c. Use of calculator, word processor, and tape recorder for home-work assignments

d. Testing modifications: extended time limits; test questions read; tests blown up to large print; tests divided into and presented in smaller parts; demonstrate mastery with less questions; use of calculator

Review/Assessment Date: _____

Participants (Name and Title):

Jane Smith, mother   Kate Jones, school counselor

John Smith, father   Dave Frank, school psychologist

Joe Brown, principal

Attachments: information regarding Section 504 of the Rehabilitation Act of 1973; Parent/Student Rights in Identification, Evaluation, and Placement.

Sample 504 Plan for an Elementary Student

ANYTOWN ELEMENTARY SCHOOL
SECTION 504 STUDENT ACCOMMODATION PLAN

Student _____ Grade __2__ DOB _____

School _____ Date of Meeting _____

1. Describe the nature of the concern:
   "Student's Name" is often unable to attend school full-time due to Chronic Fatigue Syndrome. He or she suffers from severe abdominal pain, headaches, sore throats, joint and muscle pain, and reduced stamina.

2. Describe the basis for the determination of handicap (if any):
   See attached letter from "Doctor's Name."

3. Describe how the handicap affects a major life activity:
   Interferes with regular daily school attendance and affects his or her ability to concentrate.

4. Describe the reasonable accommodations that are necessary:
   a. Home tutoring: 5 hours/week
   b. Health exempt PE
   c. Use of word processor
   d. Tutor will be provided with copies of the teachers manuals and curriculum guides and basic summaries of skills being taught.
   e. Contact will be maintained between the tutor and teachers every 2 to 4 weeks to discuss progress at home and to share activities occurring at school.
   f. "Student's Name" will be included in any class activities and have the opportunity to participate in all school activities.

Review/Assessment Date: As necessary

Participants (Name and Title):

Jane Smith, mother	Kate Jones, teacher
John Smith, father	Dave Frank, school psychologist
Joe Brown, principal	Debbie Smith, school nurse

Attachments: information regarding Section 504 of the Rehabilitation Act of 1973.

Sample IEP for a Seventh Grade YPWC

ANYTOWN CENTRAL SCHOOL
INDIVIDUALIZED EDUCATION PROGRAM

Student Information

Name _____	Student ID 111222345
Date of Birth _____	Dominant Language ___ English
Age _____	Current Grade Seventh
Sex _____	Disability Other Health Impaired
Address First Avenue	Telephone (123) 456-7890

Parent/Guardian Information

Name Smith, John	Relationship Father
Name Smith, Jame	Relationship Mother
Address First Avenue	Telephone (home) (123) 456-7890
Anytown, State 12345	Dominant Language English
	Interpreter Needed *No*

CSE Meeting Information

Committee Name ___ Anytown CSE

Type of Meeting ___ New Referral

Date of Meeting _____   Projected Annual Review* _____

Next Triennial Review _____

---

*Author's note: The annual review must be held within one year.

Least Restrictive Environment

This placement provides a program for "Student's Name" in the least restrictive environment.

Recommendations

The committee has determined that "Student's Name" is eligible to receive special education services and recommends the following:

- Special Education Programs and Related Services

Program/ Related Service	Freq. & Mins. Out of Class/ In Class	School/ District	Placement Type	Start Date End Date
CONSULTANT TEACHER SERVICES				
Consult Teach	1/wk, 60 min.	Middle School	Public School	******
Individual		Anytown District	In district	******
Consult Teach	5/wk, 600 min.	Middle School	home	******
Individual (home tutor)		Anytown District		******

- Specialized Transportation: None

- Second Language Exemption: Yes

- Test Exemptions: None

- Testing Modifications:

      Increase size of answer block
      Increase spacing
      Masks or markers to maintain place
      Reduce number of items per page
      Revised format

Calculator
Word processor
Extend time allotted to complete test
Answers recorded in any manner

- Specialized Equipment/Adaptive Devices/Assistive Technology

Calculator	Action: recommended
Word processor	Action: recommended
Books on tape	Action: recommended
Extra set of textbooks at home/ teacher's manuals for tutor	Action: recommended

- Special Alerts: Medical excuse from gym; No Physical Education

- Twelve-Month Special Service and/or Program

  July/August provider: Anytown Central School

  Math tutoring: 6 hours/wk for 8 weeks

  Location: Home

  Tutoring should consist of reinforcement of seventh grade material and preparation for eighth grade. Skills should include (******skills were listed)

Individualized Education Program Levels of Performance

Committee Decision was based on the following evaluation results, reports, and previous records:

- Psychological Levels

  Testing Date: ******WISC III
  Full Scale/Mental Processing Composite:
  Verbal/Sequential Processing:
  Performance/Simultaneous Processing:
  Achievement:

- Educational/Academic Achievement

- Social Development

  Continue to promote and encourage involvement in school activities.

- Physical Development

  Diagnosis of Chronic Fatigue Immune Dysfunction Syndrome and Orthostatic Hypotension—limits strength, vitality, and alertness.

- Management Needs

  No material resources, human resources, or environmental modifications required.

Annual Goals and Objectives*

Math Goal: The student will increase conceptual and computational skills in seventh grade mathematics.

Objectives:

1. Apply properties of irrational numbers to solve mathematical problems with 80 percent accuracy.
2. Apply concepts of percent to solve mathematical problems with 80 percent accuracy.
3. Apply knowledge of fractions to add, subtract, and write in lowest terms with 80 percent accuracy.

Evaluation Procedures: Seventh grade assignments and tests and teacher/tutor tests and observations.

Science Goal: The student will develop knowledge, concepts, and skills related to the study of astronomy.

Objectives:

1. Explain how the tilt of the Earth's axis causes seasons with 80 percent accuracy, based on teacher observation.

---

*Author note: Because of space, we have chosen to list only several of the annual goals and short-term objectives for each goal that appeared in this seventh grade YPWC's IEP. It will give you an idea of how helpful this part of the IEP can be for your child in academic planning.

2. Explain why the length of daylight changes throughout the year with 80 percent accuracy, based on teacher observation.
3. Identify the difference between a meteor, meteorite, comet, and asteroid with 80 percent accuracy, based on teacher observation.
4. Describe three principle features of each planet with 80 percent accuracy.
5. Compare and contrast Mars and Earth with 80 percent accuracy, based on teacher observation.
6. Describe the size and colors of stars and how they are born and die with 80 percent accuracy, based on teacher observation.
7. Describe the difference between solar system, galaxy, and universe with 80 percent accuracy, based on teacher observation.

Evaluation Procedures: Seventh grade assignments and tests and teacher/tutor tests and observations.

Individualized Education Program Comments

Modify curriculum and workload

Meeting Attendees

Name	**Title**
Dave Frank	School Psychologist
Joe Brown	CSE Chairperson
Jane Smith	Mother
John Smith	Father
Student Smith	Student
Kate Jones	Special Education Teacher
Jane Doe	Voting CSE Parent

Appendix I

Educational Citations

Family Education Rights and Privacy Act, 20 U.S.C.A. Section 1232g (Office of the Law Revision Council of U.S. House of Representatives, 1990).

The Inviduals with Disabilities Education Act, 20 U.S.C. Section 1400 et seq. (Office of the Law Revision Council of the U.S. House of Representatives, 1997).

The Individuals with Disabilities Education Act, "Other Health Impairment Classification" 34 C.F.R. Section 300.7 (Office of the Federal Register National Archives and Records Administration, 1997).

The Individuals with Disabilities Education Act, "IEP Meetings" 34 C.F.R. Section 300.345 (Office of the Federal Register National Archives and Records Administration, 1996).

The Individuals with Disabilities Education Act, "Content of Individualized Education Program" 34 C.F.R. Section 300.346 (Office of the Federal Register National Archives and Records Administration, 1996).

National Information Center for Children and Youth with Disabilities (NICHCY), "Questions Often Asked About Special Education Services" (NICHCY, Washington, DC: 1994).

Rehabilitation Act of 1973—Section 504, 29 U.S.C.A. Section 706(8) (Office of the Law Revision Council of U.S. House of Representatives, 1997).

Rehabilitation Act of 1973—Section 504, 34 C.F.R. Sections 104.33, 104.34, 104.35 (Office of the Federal Register National Archives and Records Administration, 1997).

* * *

You can search the U.S. Codes U.S.C. (U.S.C.A.) on the Internet at The U.S. House of Representatives Internet Law Library U.S. Code: http://law.house.gov/uscsrch.htm

You can also search the Code of Federal Regulations CFR at: http://www.access.gpo.gov/nara/cfr/cfr-retrieve.htmlpage1

Index

Tests. *See also* Mall test
  individualization of, 95, 148-149
  interpreting, 103-104
  physical environment, 103
  preparation for, 102-103
  standardized, 101-102
Throat soreness, 4, 6, 138
Toes, 4
Toys, 56
Transition services, 98, 121. *See also*
      Future plans
Transportation, to school, 80, 89
Trigger points, 6
Tutoring, at home, 98-99, 148

U.S. Codes (U.S.C.A.), 86, 87, 153
United States Department
      of Education
  Office for Civil Rights (OCR),
      90, 122
  Office of Special Education
      and Rehabilitative Services
      (OSERS), 92, 123

Unpredictability, 69-71, 78. *See also*
      Remissions and relapses

Walking, 138
Weight gain, 4, 68
Wheelchairs, 68, 138
Work world, 67, 98
World Wide Web, 16-17, 48, 49n, 117

Young person with CFIDS (YPWC)
  emotional health tips, 140-141
  and family life, 11-12, 17-18
  father's attitude, 23
  fighting diagnosis, 61-63
  independence and mobility aids,
      138-139
  information for, 54, 114-115
  outcome study, 70
  performance evaluation, 149-151
  preparation for testing, 102-103

Order Your Own Copy of
This Important Book for Your Personal Library!

A PARENTS' GUIDE TO CFIDS
How to Be an Advocate for Your Child with Chronic Fatigue Immune Dysfunction

_____ in hardbound at $39.95 (ISBN: 0-7890-0631-6)

_____ in softbound at $17.95 (ISBN: 0-7890-0711-8)

COST OF BOOKS_____

OUTSIDE USA/CANADA/
MEXICO: ADD 20%_____

POSTAGE & HANDLING_____
(US: $3.00 for first book & $1.25
for each additional book)
Outside US: $4.75 for first book
& $1.75 for each additional book)

SUBTOTAL_____

IN CANADA: ADD 7% GST_____

STATE TAX_____
(NY, OH & MN residents, please
add appropriate local sales tax)

FINAL TOTAL_____
(If paying in Canadian funds,
convert using the current
exchange rate. UNESCO
coupons welcome.)

☐ **BILL ME LATER:** ($5 service charge will be added)
(Bill-me option is good on US/Canada/Mexico orders only;
not good to jobbers, wholesalers, or subscription agencies.)

☐ Check here if billing address is different from
shipping address and attach purchase order and
billing address information.

Signature_____

☐ **PAYMENT ENCLOSED: $**_____

☐ **PLEASE CHARGE TO MY CREDIT CARD.**

☐ Visa   ☐ MasterCard   ☐ AmEx   ☐ Discover
☐ Diner's Club

Account #_____

Exp. Date_____

Signature_____

Prices in US dollars and subject to change without notice.

NAME _____

INSTITUTION _____

ADDRESS _____

CITY _____

STATE/ZIP _____

COUNTRY _____ COUNTY (NY residents only) _____

TEL _____ FAX _____

E-MAIL_____

May we use your e-mail address for confirmations and other types of information? ☐ Yes   ☐ No

Order From Your Local Bookstore or Directly From
The Haworth Press, Inc.
10 Alice Street, Binghamton, New York 13904-1580 • USA
TELEPHONE: 1-800-HAWORTH (1-800-429-6784) / Outside US/Canada: (607) 722-5857
FAX: 1-800-895-0582 / Outside US/Canada: (607) 772-6362
E-mail: getinfo@haworthpressinc.com
PLEASE PHOTOCOPY THIS FORM FOR YOUR PERSONAL USE.

BOF96

FORTHCOMING, NEW AND INFORMATIVE
BOOKS FROM THE HAWORTH MEDICAL PRESS®

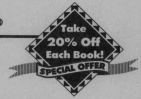
A PARENT'S GUIDE TO CFIDS
*How to Be an Advocate for Your Child
with Chronic Fatigue Immune Dysfunction Syndrome*
**David S. Bell, MD, FAAP, Mary Z. Robinson, MS,
Jean Pollard, Tom Robinson, MS, CAS,
and Bonnie Floyd, MA**
Helps you minimize the negative effects of CFIDS on
socialization and education of children afflicted with this illness
and covers situations in communicating with the doctor, the
school, and the family.
$39.95 hard. ISBN: 0-7890-0631-6.
$17.95 soft. ISBN: 0-7890-0711-8.
1999. Available now. 143 pp. with Index.
**Features treatment regimes, diagnostic criteria,
list of organizations, Web site/Internet addresses,
a glossary, and 8 appendixes.**

THE LOVE DRUG
Marching to the Beat of Ecstasy
Richard S. Cohen
*"Provides a balanced, impartial view of Ecstasy's past
and present-day history."*
—Edge Magazine
$39.95 hard. ISBN: 0-7890-0453-4.
$17.95 soft. ISBN: 0-7890-0454-2. 1998. 116 pp. with Index.
Features tables, figures, and a bibliography.

DRUGS, THE BRAIN, AND BEHAVIOR
The Pharmacology of Abuse and Dependence
**John Brick, PhD, FAPA, DABFM,
and Carlton K. Erickson, PhD**
*"Up-to-date and surprisingly readable without
'talking down' to its audience."*
—The Forensic Examiner
$49.95 hard. ISBN: 0-7890-0274-4.
$24.95 soft. ISBN: 0-7890-0275-2. 1998. 186 pp. with Index.
Features tables, figures, and diagnostic criteria.

DISEASE, PAIN,
AND SUICIDAL BEHAVIOR
*"A welcome resource for students of the complex
relationships among specific physical illnesses, pain
states, and suicidal behavior!"*
—Doody Publishing
$39.95 hard. ISBN: 0-7890-0111-X.
$14.95 soft. ISBN: 0-7890-0295-7 1997. 128 pp. with Index.
Features case studies and eight tables.

The Haworth Medical Press®
An imprint of The Haworth Press, Inc.
10 Alice Street, Binghamton, New York 13904–1580 USA

BETRAYAL BY THE BRAIN
*The Neurologic Basis of Chronic Fatigue Syndrome,
Fibromyalgia Syndrome, and Related Neural
Network Disorders*
Jay A. Goldstein, MD
*"The first giant step in addressing a neurochemical
imbalance in individuals as the cause of their maladies,
as well as the correct starting point for resolution of the
disabilities of tens of thousands of people."*
—National Association of Rehabilitation Professionals
in the Private Sector
$49.95 hard. ISBN: 1-56024-977-3.
$29.95 soft. ISBN: 1-56024-981-1. 1996. 313 pp. with Index.

Over 300 Pages!

A COMPANION VOLUME
TO DR. JAY A. GOLDSTEIN'S
BETRAYAL BY THE BRAIN
A Guide for Patients and Their Physicians
Katie Courmel
*"I picked up a copy of Betrayal by the Brain. . . . I was
able to grasp the Introduction—beyond that, he lost me.
I decided that Dr. Goldstein's work was too valuable to be
. . . inaccessible, because of its complexity, to the people
who crave an understanding of it the most—those who
suffer with CFS and FMS."*
—From the Introduction by the Author
$14.95 soft. ISBN: 0-7890-0119-5. 1996. 98 pp. with Index.

CHRONIC FATIGUE SYNDROMES
The Limbic Hypothesis
Jay A. Goldstein, MD
*"Presents what must be unrivaled clinical experience with
a condition most family doctors encounter infrequently."*
—Canadian Family Physician
$49.95 hard. ISBN: 1-56024-433-X.
$19.95 soft. ISBN: 1-56024-904-8.
1993. 259 pp. with Index.

Over 250 Pages!

THE FACTS ABOUT DRUG USE
*Coping With Drugs and Alcohol in Your Family,
at Work, in Your Community*
Barry Stimmel, MD
*"An excellent resource for identifying and
understanding drug abuse."*
—Rx Watch
$14.95 soft. ISBN: 1-56024-401-1.
1992. 374 pp. with Index.

Over 350 Pages!

POST-VIRAL FATIGUE SYNDROME
**Edited by Rachel Jenkins, MBBMRC,
and James F. Mowbray, MBB**
A reference source that provides a comprehensive account
of what is technically called myalgic encephalomyelitis (ME).
$141.95 hard. ISBN: 0-471-92846-1.
1991. 447 pp. with Index.

Over 450 Pages!

MANAGED SERVICE RESTRUCTURING IN HEALTH CARE

A Strategic Approach in a Competitive Environment

Robert L. Goldman, PhD, and Sanjib K. Mukherjee, MBA

"By following the suggested steps, services and jobs can be gainfully continued in many instances of organization restructuring."
—Abstracts of Public Administration, Development, and Environment

Selected Contents: MSR Defined • Applying Managed Service Restructuring • MSR in Practice • Reference Notes Included • Index • *more*

$39.95 hard. ISBN: 1-56024-896-3. 1995. 104 pp. with Index.

Textbooks are available for classroom adoption consideration on a 60–day examination basis. You will receive an invoice payable within 60 days along with the book. **If you decide to adopt the book, your invoice will be cancelled.** Please write to us on your institutional letterhead, indicating the textbook you would like to examine as well as the following information: course title, current text, enrollment, and decision date.

CALL OUR TOLL-FREE NUMBER: 1–800–HAWORTH
US & Canada only / 8am–5pm ET; Monday–Friday
Outside US/Canada: + 607–722–5857

FAX YOUR ORDER TO US: 1–800–895–0582
Outside US/Canada: + 607–771–0012

E-MAIL YOUR ORDER TO US:
getinfo@haworthpressinc.com

VISIT OUR WEB SITE AT:
http://www.haworthpressinc.com

Of Related Interest

IS RELIGION GOOD FOR YOUR HEALTH?

The Effects of Religion on Physical and Mental Health

Harold G. Koenig, MD

"A clear, readable overview of evidence suggesting the positive role of religion on mental and physical health."
—Religious Studies Review

$49.95 hard. ISBN: 0-7890-0166-7.
$19.95 soft. ISBN: 0-7890-0229-9. 1997. 137 pp. with Index.

WE'RE ONLINE!

Visit our online catalog and search for publications of interest to you by title, author, keyword, or subject! You'll find descriptions, reviews, and complete tables of contents of books and journals!

http://www.haworthpressinc.com

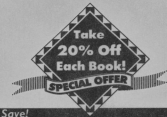

Take 20% Off Each Book! SPECIAL OFFER

Order Today and Save!

TITLE	ISBN	REGULAR PRICE	20%–OFF PRICE